The New Alpinism
TRAINING LOG

The New Alpinism Training Log

Patagonia publishes a select list of titles on wilderness, wildlife, and outdoor sports that inspire and restore a connection to the natural world.

First Edition

Disclaimer
The information provided in this book is designed to provide helpful information on the subjects covered, including endurance and strength training, and physical fitness. It is particularly designed for people who are actively participating in or would like to train for certain extreme physical activities such as rock and ice climbing.

This information is not for everyone, as many of the activities described are intense and can be dangerous. You should not undertake any of these activities unless and until you have consulted with qualified medical personnel and been cleared to participate. And, of course, if you find that you are suffering from the symptoms of any physical or medical condition, you should consult with your physician or other qualified health provider immediately. Do not avoid or disregard professional medical advice or delay in seeking it because of something you have read in this book.

All of the information contained in this book, including text, graphics, exercises, and training regimens are for informational and educational purposes only. The authors and publisher of this book shall have no liability or responsibility to any reader or any third party arising out of any injury or damage incurred as a result of the use of the information provided in this book.

Editor – John Dutton
Book Designer – Eva House
Project Manager – Jennifer Patrick
Graphic Production – Rafael Dunn, Monique Martinez
Director of Books – Karla Olson

Front Cover: Steve House leading during the first free ascent of the Italian Pillar route of Taulliraju, Cordillera Blanca, Peru. Photo by Marko Prezelj
Back Cover: Photo by Rolando Garibotti

Printed in Canada on 100 percent post-consumer recycled paper
Softcover ISBN 978-1-938340-39-0
Library of Congress Control Number 2014959034

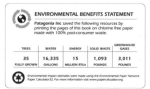

ENVIRONMENTAL BENEFITS STATEMENT
Patagonia Inc saved the following resources by printing the pages of this book on chlorine free paper made with 100% post-consumer waste.

TREES FULLY GROWN	WATER GALLONS	ENERGY MILLION BTUs	SOLID WASTE POUNDS	GREENHOUSE GASES POUNDS
35	16,335	15	1,093	3,011

Environmental impact estimates were made using the Environmental Paper Network Paper Calculator 3.2. For more information visit www.papercalculator.org.

1%
FOR THE
PLANET
MEMBER

One percent of the sales from this book go to the preservation and restoration of the natural environment.

The New Alpinism
TRAINING LOG

Steve House and Scott Johnston

patagonia®

THE NEW ALPINISM TRAINING LOG

Personal Information

Name   _____

Street   _____

City   _____

Country   _____

Telephone   _____

Email   _____

What is a mountain? An obstacle; a transcendence; above all, an effect.
Salman Rushdie

TRAIN SMART

The concept of stress followed by recovery underlies the training effect that *Training for the New Alpinism* is based on. The chart below graphically illustrates that concept. It drives home the point that training actually makes you weaker and that it is during recovery that you become fitter. Heed this simple idea and pay attention to how well recovered you are before undertaking the next workout, and you can build fitness consistently over many months. Force your body to endure stress levels it is unprepared for or allow insufficient recovery time after training sessions, and you will struggle to adapt to the training.

P 74-75

Recovery and Supercompensation

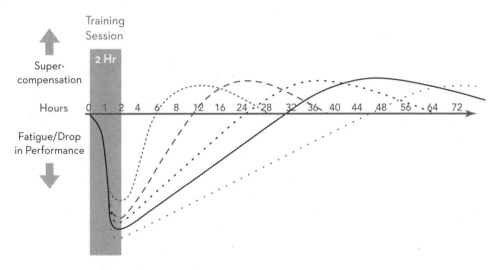

. . . . At or Below the Aerobic Threshold: **Zones 1 & 2**
– – – – – Between Aerobic Threshold and the Lactate Threshold: **Zone 3**
. . . . Above Lactate Threshold: **Zone 4**
————— Maximal Intensity: **Zone 5**
. . . . Strength Training

Recovery and supercompensation times after a two-hour session of various intensities. The vertical scale is purely qualitative, but the horizontal scale is in hours. While there is some interpersonal variability to these numbers, the originator of this scale collected data on hundreds of swimmers over many years to arrive at these values. It has been your authors' experience that these values hold quite well. Reproduced from *The Science of Winning* by Jan Olbrecht, courtesy of F&G Partners Publishing.

PREFACE

The value of the training log

I used to think I was training. In 1994, I was preparing for my second Himalayan expedition, a lightweight attempt on the beautiful Thalay Sagar. I was working as a mountain guide, teaching snow, ice, and glacier skills six out of every seven days. After work—we were camped on the moraine—I'd run four miles down to the van, and back. On my one free day per week, I'd boulder along the train tracks, frustrated at my lack of rock-climbing fitness. Our journey to colorful India, and through the mountains, was vivid—the memories still burn in my mind's eye. Yet our climb did not go well. We packed too light and nearly froze at 20,000 feet on our first attempt. The next morning we rappelled, taking an entire day to do what should have been a fast descent.

In 2003, I started to work with my first coach, and she gave me my first training log: a primitive, but practical, spreadsheet with columns for different training activities and heart-rate zones. This was my first taste of real training: daily workouts, keeping to a schedule, powering through the hard weeks, and feeling guilty and lazy on the easy weeks. Unfortunately, her training plan, and my inexperience, caused me to blow up and after a few months I became deathly ill. The next year I began working with Scott Johnston, and his coaching over the next dozen years was instrumental in every climb I succeeded on. He taught me most of what I know about training, first as an athlete, and now as an author and teacher in my own right.

Through all of these years I kept using those original log pages, the photocopies getting fainter and fainter each year. Those same pages are used as the templates for the Annual and Weekly Training Logs that appear on pages 185–186 of *Training for the New Alpinism*. The book you now hold has taken updates of those time-tested tables and married them with the material from *Training for the New Alpinism*. What you hold is not a log, it's a personalized guide: it's *Training for the New Alpinism*, distilled, organized, and translated into a flowchart so that you, with the original book, can efficiently plan and execute real training.

P 185–186

Go simply. Train smart. Climb well.

STEVE HOUSE
Ridgway, Colorado
September 2014

INTRODUCTION

Getting the most from this book

This logbook is written as a companion to *Training for the New Alpinism*. You will need to use that book as a reference both in laying out the training plans herein and during the training process.

P 47-49

To maximize enjoyment and success in your training, you'll want to have a goal and a clear plan to reach that goal. Along with climbing, lifting weights, and running, successful training involves the management of numerous tasks on a short-, medium-, and long-term basis. In order to succeed you have to comply with the three cardinal principles of training: Continuity, Gradualness, and Modulation (see pages 47–49 in *Training for the New Alpinism*). We'll start by sketching out a plan that acknowledges and incorporates both your training tasks as well as family and work responsibilities.

WHAT IS TRAINING?

Training for climbing is best thought of as exercise planned and executed with the aim of producing improvements in the physical and mental qualities that athletes need to complete their climbs. To this end, training requires:

- **An intelligent plan** that incorporates a gradual increase in training load that fluctuates between training stress and recovery so that your body's natural supercompensation can take effect (see pages 46-47 in *Training for the New Alpinism*).

P 46-47

- **A constant evaluation** of the training effect (felt as fatigue) and recovery (feeling rested) to mindfully implement modifications to the plan as needed.

Examples of the Training Effect

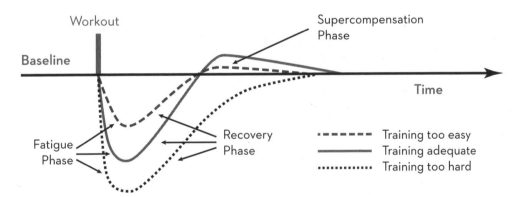

Long-Term Training Effect

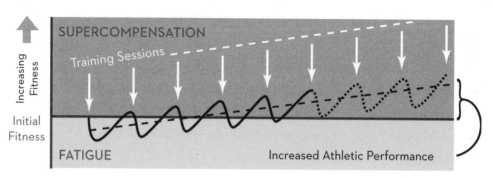

THIS BOOK WILL GUIDE YOU TO

P 66–72

- **Establish realistic climbing goals** that keep you motivated and focused on the long term when weather, illness, injury, or common laziness is holding you back.

- **Lay out an annual (or seasonal) plan** that lets you visualize the big picture of what you hope to accomplish.

- **From that annual plan** you'll work backward to develop the periodized structure we discuss in *Training for the New Alpinism* (see pages 66–72). The purpose and advantage of establishing periods is that you have easily comprehensible short-term training goals so you can narrow your focus to dealing with the most important tasks.

KEY IDEAS TO REMEMBER

- **Plan only one period at a time.** Wait until you are nearly finished with the current period before starting to plan the next period. Be sure to write into the plan upcoming significant events like travel, family commitments, or other planned breaks in training as you learn of them to maximize your success in working around known obligations.

- **After laying out each period plan,** you will construct weekly plans that fit the actual workouts that need to be accomplished during that period. The log section will give you further guidance. You'll need to fit these around the rest of your life: your family, job, school, etc. Assign workouts to certain days of the week and try to adhere to this. We find that athletes do well with a schedule. Obviously things will not always work out perfectly and you need to be flexible; under no circumstance is it a good idea to try to make up for lost workouts by cramming them into an otherwise full schedule. If something gets in the way, be it weather, job, illness, or an unexpected visit to your kid's principal's office, you need to recognize that you cannot make up for lost training time. Keep moving forward.

- **We find it easiest to make a detailed plan** not more than two to four weeks ahead so that you can ensure that things can be adjusted to fit in with the realities of life.

- **Record what you *actually* do in the logbook area.** This section is essentially a diary where you record what you did in terms of volume, intensity, and type of training.

- **Climbing notes.** We've provided a space for you to record your climbing as it relates to your training. Time spent climbing is the most important metric to record, but we've also allowed space for recording the route grades and number of pitches climbed.

- **Workout notes.** The most important record keeping you will do is to write how you felt during each activity. We provide a place to enter the letter grade for each workout (as described in chapter 2 of *Training for the New Alpinism*), along with a sizable space to record notes. We recommend recording things like your perceptions of your fitness,

Chapter 2

fatigue, and times for workouts. This will allow you to look back weeks or months later and see trends. Careful note taking will allow you to see what you did leading into that month and where you were killing it every time you went out. Perhaps even more importantly, it will allow you some insight into understanding training mistakes that lead to excess fatigue or sickness. These notes tell the story of your progress; don't shortcut them.

WHAT YOU WILL WRITE IN THE PLAN

In the annual plan you will write big-picture things:

- **Total target training hours** for the year.

- **Forecasted, progressive training hours.**

- **Layouts of two- to three-week progressions** with recovery weeks built in at least every four weeks. We'll remind you of this in the log.

- **Climbing trips and known breaks** in training. For instance, you're headed to Louisiana for a family Christmas: no hills, no climbing to be found. Designate that as a recovery week and work backward, plan the training leading into it so you can relax and enjoy mom's cooking.

Then, in each weekly plan take out the microscope and look at what you can fit in and when. Be realistic. You are the coach now and need to fit workouts in where you can. Have at least one full day off from training each week to allow a day to get caught up on life.

WHAT YOU WILL RECORD IN THE LOG

Be honest in your recording. This means if you spent four hours at the crag but only climbed three pitches, don't write four hours in the climbing column for that day. Chances are good you actually climbed for forty-five minutes. Be consistent. If you are going to record time spent doing yoga or stretching (which is a fine thing to do), then do it every time. This is meant to be a record for you to refer back to. Accuracy will give you the best feedback months later when your memory of that workout fades. The feedback you get from an accurate training log will be the best guide for laying out future training plans. Take solace knowing that the first training cycle is the most difficult to plan because your learning curve is steep.

Aerobic Training

In the columns headed Z1, Z2, and Z3 (see chapter 2 in *Training for the New Alpinism*), you'll record the time spent in each respective heart-rate (HR) zone; the modality is not as important. In winter and spring you may be doing a lot of ski touring. In the summer and fall you may be doing mostly trail running and approaches to alpine climbs. Don't lose sleep over recording the precise minutes per any particular zone; that level of accuracy is simply not necessary. Many recording HR monitors and GPS devices allow you to download the file for each workout into a training log program. That data can then be manipulated in many ways. These are fine tools for dedicated athletes who especially love gadgets, but they are not necessary to keep good records. Even using a HR monitor is optional if you have a good sense of your aerobic threshold, or AeT (see pages 60–61 in *Training for the New Alpinism*). For the vast majority of this training you should aim to stay in Zone 1 or Zone 2. Knowing what your breathing feels and sounds like during this training may be all the feedback you need. Be consistent in both your training and recording.

Strength

We have provided two places to record the strength training work that you do. The first is a single column in the weekly log chart where you record the length of time of each workout. The second place is a separate chart specific

Chapter 2

P 60-61

to each period's strength training workouts. In this chart you can record the sets, reps, and resistance for the various exercises. This system allows you to see the progress you are making through that period.

Workout Notes

We have allowed considerable space for you to write in notes about your workout. Add in notes like the name of the trail you ran or the peak you bagged. You might also want to write down how you slept afterward if it was unusual. This is also a place you can record upcoming events that will affect your training time, such as an upcoming deadline at work, final exams, or attending Uncle Harry's fourth wedding.

Workout Grades

Each day has a place for you to grade that workout. We have long used:

- **A** I felt like superman!

- **B** Good workout.

- **C** I felt flat today.

- **D** I had to modify the workout.

- **E** I couldn't complete the workout.

Climbing

We have provided space for recording the number of pitches of climbing you did as well as the amount of time spent climbing. Generally we have found it useful to record both as this can easily correlate to specific routes. For example, if you are training for the Moonflower Buttress of Mount Hunter, essentially a thirty-six-pitch ice climb, then knowing that your biggest climbing day in the nine months preceding your departure for Alaska was six pitches will explain your failure. If your goal climb involves a specific number of technical pitches, you'll have the option of using the pitch-per-day total as another measure of relative volume.

When recording time, we find it most useful to record only the actual amount of time spent climbing. We don't count belaying time. It's okay to estimate: if you're top-roping at a sport crag you're familiar with, ten to fifteen minutes per pitch might be about right. For a remote alpine climb you can record the approach and return in the appropriate Zone 1 or Zone 2 columns. If there is some third-class scrambling, then by all means include this also in these endurance zone columns. Then record the climbing time (minus breaks for belays or lunch on the summit) in the climbing column. You needn't use a stopwatch to calculate each pitch's time. Instead, a good estimate of climbing time, if you are swinging leads and belaying, is that you are pretty inactive for half the time the climb takes. So if a long alpine route takes eight hours you can record four hours of climbing time. If on a long mountaineering route where you are on the move all day with only short breaks of less than fifteen minutes, you can log the entire climbing time.

SELF-ASSESSMENT

Open your computer, set a timer, and write nonstop for ten minutes about your strengths and weaknesses both in climbing and in life—they are often related. Putting this awareness front and center will help you plot an effective course to get to where you want to go. Successful self-management is predicated on self-awareness.

Let's take a look at a hypothetical example of a climber with a goal of climbing the Cassin Ridge on Denali. The Cassin Ridge is a big route on a big mountain with serious consequences if something goes wrong. Logistics, weather, fitness, climbing skill, acclimatization, glacier travel (both on and off skis), and winter camping skills will all play major roles in the outcome.

This hypothetical climber will first need to do an honest assessment of all the components that will go into making this climb successful. Is he fit enough? How fast can she move while carrying four to five days of food and gear? Does he have sufficient climbing skills? Has she spent multiple nights out in winter conditions? Does he know how much food to purchase and pack? Is she strong at altitude? Is he comfortable with skiing on glaciers while wearing a big pack?

After this assessment process you should know where you need to focus to give yourself the best chance of success. While some areas like logistics, winter camping, or skiing skills are not going to be directly addressed in the training plan, it is a good idea to make note of them in the assessment. Where this log will be most useful is helping you deal with the fitness aspect of your preparation for your goal.

Goal setting is far from simply stating an outcome you hope for, such as the Cassin Ridge. Dreams are wonderful inspiration, but self-assessment and self-management are critical to making the leap from dream to reality.

ALPINE COMBINE

Now is the time to get down to the sweaty part. This test will help give you some perspective and a baseline on your general state of physical fitness. Don't be discouraged if you have some deficiencies. It is far easier—and more effective—to improve your weaknesses than it is to boost your strengths. Please see pages 176–179 in *Training for the New Alpinism*.

P 176–179

You'll notice that the first and perhaps most relevant test is the vertical hike test. You can choose to do this on a nearby steep mountain slope or, as we suggest for repeatability, use a box to step up and down. The reason we place such emphasis on this test is that it does a fairly good job of modeling the specific demands of climbing a steep slope, which even the most technical alpine climbs usually have in abundance.

We have set up a reporting survey for the Alpine Combine. To have your results included in a future edition of *Training for the New Alpinism*, visit: https://www.surveymonkey.com/s/x9srp6v.

ALPINE COMBINE TEST

Date	6 /26 /22.	__ / __ / __	__ / __ / __
Exercise	**Time/Reps**	**Time/Reps**	**Time/Reps**
1000' Climb or Box Step-Ups	1500+ 38 min. 1,000/20		
Dips in 60 Seconds			
Sit-Ups in 60 Seconds			
Pull-Ups in 60 Seconds			
Box Jumps in 60 Seconds			
Push-Ups in 60 Seconds			

ANNUAL TRAINING PLANNING

Painting the big picture

For those who have been through this process already and know how many annual training hours you completed last year, you can simply begin the Transition Period with 50 percent of the previous year's average.

P 189

If you're not sure how much volume to start with, you need to arrive at a reasonable estimate for the number of hours to train. Study page 189 of *Training for the New Alpinism* and use the table and guidelines there.

If you have been training at a high level for several years you'll want to limit your yearly training volume increase to between 5 and 10 percent. If you're in the first two to four years of following an organized training plan, then you may be able to increase your training volume from year to year by 10 to even 25 percent. Regardless of which situation you are in, make this determination based upon last year's volume and how you handled that.

We recommend you use a pencil when filling out the Annual Training Plan. We want to remind you that this annual planning process is meant to create a guide, not a commandment handed down from on high.

SAMPLE PLAN

Week	Period	Event	Planned Hours	Suggested Volume Increase on Previous Week	Completed Hours
1	Transition	Alpine Combine Test		0	
2	Transition	AeT Nose Breathing Test, Page 57		0	
3	Transition	General Conditioning Workouts		0	
4	Transition			+10%	
5	Transition			+10%	
6	Transition			+5%	
7	Transition	Alpine Combine Retest		+5%	
8	Transition	AeT Nose Breathing Test		Drop 50%	
1	Base	1 RM Test, Page 229		+10% of Transition Week 7	
2	Base	Capacity Building Workouts		+10% to 20%	
3	Base			+10% to 20%	
4	Base			-25% to -30%	
5	Base			Same as Base Week 3	
6	Base			0%	
7	Base			+25%	
8	Base			-50%	
9	Base			Same as Base Week 7	
10	Base			+5% to 10%	
11	Base			+5% to 10%	
12	Base			-50%	
13	Base			Same as Base Week 11	
14	Base			0%	

Week	Period	Strength	Page References *Training for the New Alpinism*
1	Transition	General & Core	Start with a volume of 50% of last year's weekly average. See pages 188-191.
2	Transition	General & Core	See pages 192-206 for core strength info. See pages 207-221 for general strength info.
3	Transition	General & Core	
4	Transition	General & Core	
5	Transition	General & Core	
6	Transition	General & Core	
7	Transition	General & Core	
8	Transition	General & Core	
1	Base	Core & Max	Calculate based on completed hours, not planned hours.
2	Base	Core & Max	See pages 226-232 for Max Strength info. See pages 241-253 for Base Period planning info.
3	Base	Core & Max	
4	Base	Core & Max	
5	Base	Core & Max	
6	Base	Core & Max	
7	Base	Core & Max	
8	Base	Core & Max	
9	Base	Muscular Endurance & Max	See pages 233-241 for Muscular Endurance info.
10	Base	Muscular Endurance & Max	
11	Base	Muscular Endurance & Max	
12	Base	Muscular Endurance & Max	
13	Base	Muscular Endurance & Max	
14	Base	Muscular Endurance & Max	

SAMPLE PLAN

Week	Period	Event	Planned Hours	Suggested Volume Increase on Previous Week	Completed Hours
15	Base			+20%	
16	Base			-50% to -70%	
17	Base			Same as Base Week 15	
18	Base			-25%	
19	Base			Same as Base Week 17	
20	Base			0%	
1	Specific	Training Mimics Goal Climb		80% of Last Base Week	
2	Specific	Training Mimics Goal Climb		Drop 10%	
3	Specific	Training Mimics Goal Climb		0%	
4	Specific	Training Mimics Goal Climb		0%	
1	Taper	No Hard Workouts		Drop 50%	
2	Taper	No Hard Workouts		Drop 20%	
1	Peak	Goal Period Climbs			
2	Peak				
3	Peak				
4	Peak				
5	Peak	Return to Base Training		Same as Middle of Base Period	
6	Peak	Return to Base Training		0%	
7	Peak	Return to Base Training		0%	
8	Peak				
9	Peak				
10	Peak				

Week	Period	Strength	Page References *Training for the New Alpinism*
15	Base	Muscular Endurance & Max	
16	Base	Muscular Endurance & Max	
17	Base	Muscular Endurance	
18	Base	Muscular Endurance & Max	
19	Base	Muscular Endurance	
20	Base	Muscular Endurance & Max	
1	Specific	Max Maintenance	See pages 255–271 for Specific Period planning info.
2	Specific	Max Maintenance	
3	Specific	Max Maintenance	
4	Specific	Max Maintenance	
1	Taper	Max Maintenance	See pages 273–279 for Taper and Peak info.
2	Taper	Max Maintenance	
1	Peak		Your peak fitness of the year should last about four weeks without returning to training.
2	Peak		
3	Peak		
4	Peak		
5	Peak	Max	Refer to page 275 on how to prolong Peak Period.
6	Peak	Max	
7	Peak	Max	
8	Peak		
9	Peak		
10	Peak		

ANNUAL TRAINING PLAN

DATE _____ / _____ / _____ to _____ / _____ / _____

Week	Period	Event	Planned Hours	Suggested Volume Increase on Previous Week	Completed Hours
1	Transition				
2	Transition				
3	Transition				
4	Transition				
5	Transition				
6	Transition				
7	Transition				
8	Transition				
1	Base				
2	Base				
3	Base				
4	Base				
5	Base				
6	Base				
7	Base				
8	Base				
9	Base				
10	Base				
11	Base				
12	Base				
13	Base				
14	Base				

Week	Period	Strength	Page References *Training for the New Alpinism*
1	Transition		
2	Transition		
3	Transition		
4	Transition		
5	Transition		
6	Transition		
7	Transition		
8	Transition		
1	Base		
2	Base		
3	Base		
4	Base		
5	Base		
6	Base		
7	Base		
8	Base		
9	Base		
10	Base		
11	Base		
12	Base		
13	Base		
14	Base		

ANNUAL TRAINING PLAN

DATE ____ / ____ / ____ to ____ / ____ / ____

Week	Period	Event	Planned Hours	Suggested Volume Increase on Previous Week	Completed Hours
15	Base				
16	Base				
17	Base				
18	Base				
19	Base				
20	Base				
1	Specific				
2	Specific				
3	Specific				
4	Specific				
1	Taper				
2	Taper				
1	Peak				
2	Peak				
3	Peak				
4	Peak				
5	Peak				
6	Peak				
7	Peak				
8	Peak				
9	Peak				
10	Peak				

Week	Period	Strength	Page References *Training for the New Alpinism*
15	Base		
16	Base		
17	Base		
18	Base		
19	Base		
20	Base		
1	Specific		
2	Specific		
3	Specific		
4	Specific		
1	Taper		
2	Taper		
1	Peak		
2	Peak		
3	Peak		
4	Peak		
5	Peak		
6	Peak		
7	Peak		
8	Peak		
9	Peak		
10	Peak		

DATE ____ / ____ / ____ to ____ / ____ / ____

Week	Period	Altitude +/-	# of Pitches	Time in Rec/Z 1	Time in Z 2	Time in Z 3	Time for Strength
1	Transition						
2	Transition						
3	Transition						
4	Transition						
5	Transition						
6	Transition						
7	Transition						
8	Transition						
1	Base						
2	Base						
3	Base						
4	Base						
5	Base						
6	Base						
7	Base						
8	Base						
9	Base						
10	Base						
11	Base						
12	Base						
13	Base						
14	Base						
Subtotal							

Week	Period	Altitude +/-	# of Pitches	Time in Rec/Z 1	Time in Z 2	Time in Z 3	Time for Strength
15	Base						
16	Base						
17	Base						
18	Base						
19	Base						
20	Base						
1	Specific						
2	Specific						
3	Specific						
4	Specific						
1	Taper						
2	Taper						
1	Peak						
2	Peak						
3	Peak						
4	Peak						
5	Peak						
6	Peak						
7	Peak						
8	Peak						
9	Peak						
10	Peak						
Grand Total							

TRANSITION PERIOD PLANNING

Are you fit enough to train?

These weeks are meant to transition you back into training after an extended break. Your mind and body need some time to get into athlete mode. If you're like us, your motivation will be very high at the beginning of a new training cycle, so stick to the plan even when it feels too easy (as it probably will). It is easy to write big numbers on paper, but if you come out of the gate too hard you'll have difficulty in maintaining the progression later on. We recommend that you study pages 68 and 188–194 of *Training for the New Alpinism* to understand what you're doing in this period.

Refer to the Annual Training Plan worksheet as a starting point to fill out the first three weeks of the Transition Period plan that follows.

P 68 & P 188–194

NOTES FOR WEEKS 1–3

- **Plan one Zone 1 workout** that comprises 25 percent of your total weekly aerobic volume.

- **Plan one Zone 2 aerobic session** (exercising at the top of conversational pace) that comprises 10 percent of your total weekly aerobic volume.

- **Plan two General Strength sessions** each week; use Scott's Killer Core Routine as a warm-up.

- **Make up any remaining volume** with easy aerobic exercise at Zone 1 or recovery pace.

- **Climb one day.** Do a minimum of five to six pitches one to two number grades below your current top ability. Note that if climbing skill is preventing you from achieving your goals you may climb up to three times a week. Substitute this climbing time for the Zone 2 and any remaining Zone 1 volume left after the one long workout of the week.

Once you have completed several weeks of training, you're ready to plan the upcoming weeks. We find it handy to plan two weeks in advance.

NOTES FOR WEEKS 4–5

- **Repeat all the same workouts** as week 3, but increase volume by 10 percent each week.

- **Climb one day.** Do a minimum of five or six pitches one to two number grades below your current top ability. Note that if climbing skill is preventing you from achieving your goals you may climb up to three times a week. Substitute this climbing time for the Zone 2 and any remaining Zone 1 volume left after the one long workout of the week.

NOTES FOR WEEKS 6–7

- **Repeat all the same workouts** as week 5 but increase volume by 5 percent each week.

- **Climb one day.** Do a minimum of six to eight pitches one to two number grades below your current top ability. If climbing skill is preventing you from achieving your goals, you may climb up to three times a week. Substitute this climbing time for the Zone 2 and any remaining Zone 1 volume left after the one long workout of the week.

NOTES FOR WEEK 8

- **Drop volume by 50 percent** of week 7 and do shorter versions of the same workouts.

- **Climb no more than one day,** five pitches one number grade below your top ability.

- **This is a consolidation week** and it should feel easy.

As you get used to using this new log, be sure to make good use of the notes section. If you've been gradual in your progression during these eight weeks, you should feel noticeably fitter than when you started and fired up to move into the meat of the training during the Base Period.

DATE ____ / ____ / ____ to ____ / ____ / ____

> **!** This week's aerobic training volume should be approximately 50% of your average weekly volume for the past training year. Supplement with the general and core strength programs.
>
> P 183–221

WEEKLY TRAINING LOG

Activity by Time	Climb	Approach	Run	____	____	Altitude + / -	Time in Rec/Z 1	Time in Z 2	Time in Z 3	Time for Strength
M Plan										
Completed										
T Plan										
Completed										
W Plan										
Completed										
Th Plan										
Completed										
F Plan										
Completed										
S Plan										
Completed										
Su Plan										
Completed										

Target Hours This Week	
Actual Hours This Week	
Cumulative Training Hours	

> The most important metric to record in your climbing is time. During this week try to climb at least 5-6 pitches that are 1-2 number grades below your current redpoint ability. When you climb alpine routes, record total time and the grade of the most difficult pitch.

CLIMBING NOTES

Date	__ / __ / __	__ / __ / __	__ / __ / __
Vertical Gain			
Grades			
# of Pitches			

STRENGTH TRAINING

Core Routine	_ / _ / _		_ / _ / _	
Exercise	Reps	Weight	Reps	Weight
Strict Sit-Ups				
Bird Dogs				
Windshield Wipers				
3-P/2-Point Planks				
Kayakers				
Super Push-Ups				
Hanging Leg Raises				
Bridges				
Gymnast L-Sits				
Side Planks				

General Strength Routine	_ / _ / _		_ / _ / _	
Exercise	Reps	Weight	Reps	Weight
TGUs				
Split Squats				
Push-Ups				
Box Step-Ups				
Dips				
Squats				
Pull-Ups*				
Wall-Facing Squats				
Isometric Hangs*				

* Starred exercises are for climbers with technical climbing objectives.

Do Scott's Killer Core Routine **once** through with 30 seconds between exercises. See appendix for illustrations.

If you can do more than 10 reps or hold a pose longer than 10 seconds, add resistance for more challenge. Aim to achieve maximum core tension and hold perfect form rather than do more reps.

P 192–206

Complete circuit **once** in each workout.

Complete a max of 10 reps of each.

Do not go to failure on these sets.

30 seconds' rest between exercises.

Focus on doing these exercises with good form.

P 207–221

WEEKLY WORKOUT NOTES

	Grade	Workout Notes
M		
T		
W		
Th		
F		
S		
Su		

TRANSITION PERIOD

DATE _____/_____/_____ to _____/_____/_____

> **!** This week's aerobic training volume should be equal to last week's completed training volume. Complete both the general and core strength programs.

 P 183–221

WEEKLY TRAINING LOG

Activity by Time		Climb	Approach	Run	____	____	Altitude +/-	Time in Rec/Z 1	Time in Z 2	Time in Z 3	Time for Strength
M	Plan										
	Completed										
T	Plan										
	Completed										
W	Plan										
	Completed										
Th	Plan										
	Completed										
F	Plan										
	Completed										
S	Plan										
	Completed										
Su	Plan										
	Completed										

Target Hours This Week	
Actual Hours This Week	
Cumulative Training Hours	

 During this week try to climb a minimum of 5–6 pitches that are 1–2 number grades below your current redpoint ability. Resist the temptation to increase the time spent climbing by more than 5–10% per week.

CLIMBING NOTES

Date	__/__/__					__/__/__					__/__/__				
Vertical Gain															
Grades															
# of Pitches															

STRENGTH TRAINING

Core Routine	_ / _ / _		_ / _ / _	
Exercise	Reps	Weight	Reps	Weight
Strict Sit-Ups				
Bird Dogs				
Windshield Wipers				
3-P/2-Point Planks				
Kayakers				
Super Push-Ups				
Hanging Leg Raises				
Bridges				
Gymnast L-Sits				
Side Planks				

General Strength Routine	_ / _ / _		_ / _ / _	
Exercise	Reps	Weight	Reps	Weight
TGUs				
Split Squats				
Push-Ups				
Box Step-Ups				
Dips				
Squats				
Pull-Ups*				
Wall-Facing Squats				
Isometric Hangs*				

* Starred exercises are for climbers with technical climbing objectives.

Do Scott's Killer Core Routine **once** through with 30 seconds between exercises. See appendix for illustrations.

If you can do more than 10 reps or hold a pose longer than 10 seconds, add resistance for more challenge. Aim to achieve maximum core tension and hold perfect form rather than do more reps.

P 192–206

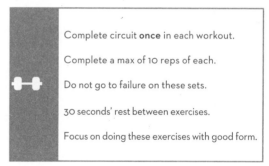

Complete circuit **once** in each workout.

Complete a max of 10 reps of each.

Do not go to failure on these sets.

30 seconds' rest between exercises.

Focus on doing these exercises with good form.

P 207–221

WEEKLY WORKOUT NOTES

	Grade	Workout Notes
M		
T		
W		
Th		
F		
S		
Su		

DATE ____ / ____ / ____ to ____ / ____ / ____

> **!** Maintain the same completed training volume as last week. You should be feeling ready to add more volume by now; this is normal and good. Patience now will pay dividends later.
>
> P 183–221

WEEKLY TRAINING LOG

Activity by Time	Climb	Approach	Run	___	___	Altitude +/-	Time in Rec/Z 1	Time in Z 2	Time in Z 3	Time for Strength
M Plan										
Completed										
T Plan										
Completed										
W Plan										
Completed										
Th Plan										
Completed										
F Plan										
Completed										
S Plan										
Completed										
Su Plan										
Completed										

Target Hours This Week

Actual Hours This Week

Cumulative Training Hours

> During this week try to climb a minimum of 5–6 pitches that are 1–2 number grades below your current redpoint ability. Resist the temptation to increase the time spent climbing by more than 5–10% per week.

CLIMBING NOTES

Date	_/_/_					_/_/_					_/_/_				
Vertical Gain															
Grades															
# of Pitches															

STRENGTH TRAINING

Core Routine	__/__/__		__/__/__	
Exercise	Reps	Weight	Reps	Weight
Strict Sit-Ups	/	/	/	/
Bird Dogs	/	/	/	/
Windshield Wipers	/	/	/	/
3-P/2-Point Planks	/	/	/	/
Kayakers	/	/	/	/
Super Push-Ups	/	/	/	/
Hanging Leg Raises	/	/	/	/
Bridges	/	/	/	/
Gymnast L-Sits	/	/	/	/
Side Planks	/	/	/	/

General Strength Routine	__/__/__		__/__/__	
Exercise	Reps	Weight	Reps	Weight
TGUs	/	/	/	/
Split Squats	/	/	/	/
Push-Ups	/	/	/	/
Box Step-Ups	/	/	/	/
Dips	/	/	/	/
Squats	/	/	/	/
Pull-Ups*	/	/	/	/
Wall-Facing Squats	/	/	/	/
Isometric Hangs*	/	/	/	/

* Starred exercises are for climbers with technical climbing objectives.

Do this routine **twice** through with 30 seconds between exercises. If you can do more than 10 reps or hold a pose longer than 10 seconds, add resistance for more challenge. Aim to achieve maximum core tension and hold perfect form rather than do more reps. By this time you should be familiarized with the core routine. Drop exercises that are too easy. Concentrate on your weaknesses.

P 192–206

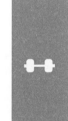

Complete circuit **twice** in each workout.

Complete a max of 10 reps of each.

Do not go to failure on these sets.

30 seconds' rest between exercises.

Focus on doing these exercises with good form.

P 207–221

WEEKLY WORKOUT NOTES

	Grade	Workout Notes
M		
T		
W		
Th		
F		
S		
Su		

DATE _____ / _____ / _____ to _____ / _____ / _____

> **!** This week's aerobic training volume should be approximately 10% more than what you completed in week 3. You can do the same workouts as last week, but with a slight increase in volume. Continue with the general and core strength programs.
>
> P 183-221

WEEKLY TRAINING LOG

Activity by Time	Climb	Approach	Run	____	____	Altitude + / -	Time in Rec/Z 1	Time in Z 2	Time in Z 3	Time for Strength
M Plan										
Completed										
T Plan										
Completed										
W Plan										
Completed										
Th Plan										
Completed										
F Plan										
Completed										
S Plan										
Completed										
Su Plan										
Completed										

Target Hours This Week	
Actual Hours This Week	
Cumulative Training Hours	

> During this week try to climb a minimum of 5-6 pitches that are 1-2 number grades below your current redpoint ability.

CLIMBING NOTES

Date	_/_/_	_/_/_	_/_/_
Vertical Gain			
Grades			
# of Pitches			

STRENGTH TRAINING

Core Routine	__/__/__		__/__/__	
Exercise	Reps	Weight	Reps	Weight
Strict Sit-Ups	/	/	/	/
Bird Dogs	/	/	/	/
Windshield Wipers	/	/	/	/
3-P/2-Point Planks	/	/	/	/
Kayakers	/	/	/	/
Super Push-Ups	/	/	/	/
Hanging Leg Raises	/	/	/	/
Bridges	/	/	/	/
Gymnast L-Sits	/	/	/	/
Side Planks	/	/	/	/

General Strength Routine	__/__/__		__/__/__	
Exercise	Reps	Weight	Reps	Weight
TGUs	/	/	/	/
Split Squats	/	/	/	/
Push-Ups	/	/	/	/
Box Step-Ups	/	/	/	/
Dips	/	/	/	/
Squats	/	/	/	/
Pull-Ups*	/	/	/	/
Wall-Facing Squats	/	/	/	/
Isometric Hangs*	/	/	/	/

* Starred exercises are for climbers with technical climbing objectives.

Do this routine **twice** through with 30 seconds between exercises. If you can do more than 10 reps or hold a pose longer than 10 seconds, add resistance for more challenge. Aim to achieve maximum core tension and hold perfect form rather than do more reps. By this time you should be familiarized with the core routine. Drop exercises that are too easy. Concentrate on your weaknesses.

P 192–206

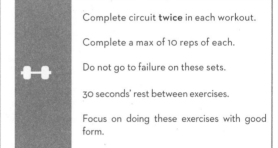

Complete circuit **twice** in each workout.

Complete a max of 10 reps of each.

Do not go to failure on these sets.

30 seconds' rest between exercises.

Focus on doing these exercises with good form.

P 207–221

WEEKLY WORKOUT NOTES

	Grade	Workout Notes
M		
T		
W		
Th		
F		
S		
Su		

TRANSITION PERIOD

DATE _____/_____/_____ to _____/_____/_____

 This week's aerobic training volume should be approximately 10% more than what you completed in week 4. Again, you may copy the previous week's workouts, with added volume. Keep doing the valuable general and core strength programs **twice** a week.

 P 183-221

WEEKLY TRAINING LOG

Activity by Time		Climb	Approach	Run	____	____	Altitude +/-	Time in Rec/Z1	Time in Z2	Time in Z3	Time for Strength
M	Plan										
	Completed										
T	Plan										
	Completed										
W	Plan										
	Completed										
Th	Plan										
	Completed										
F	Plan										
	Completed										
S	Plan										
	Completed										
Su	Plan										
	Completed										

Target Hours This Week

Actual Hours This Week

Cumulative Training Hours

 During this week try to climb a minimum of 5-6 pitches that are 1-2 number grades below your current redpoint ability.

CLIMBING NOTES

Date	__/__/__	__/__/__	__/__/__
Vertical Gain			
Grades			
# of Pitches			

TRANSITION

STRENGTH TRAINING

Core Routine	_/_/_		_/_/_	
Exercise	Reps	Weight	Reps	Weight
Strict Sit-Ups	/	/	/	/
Bird Dogs	/	/	/	/
Windshield Wipers	/	/	/	/
3-P/2-Point Planks	/	/	/	/
Kayakers	/	/	/	/

Core Routine				
Exercise	Reps	Weight	Reps	Weight
Super Push-Ups	/	/	/	/
Hanging Leg Raises	/	/	/	/
Bridges	/	/	/	/
Gymnast L-Sits	/	/	/	/
Side Planks	/	/	/	/

 Do this routine **twice** through with 30 seconds between exercises.

 P 192–206

General Strength Routine	_/_/_		_/_/_	
Exercise	Reps	Weight	Reps	Weight
TGUs	/ /	/ /	/ /	/ /
Split Squats	/ /	/ /	/ /	/ /
Push-Ups	/ /	/ /	/ /	/ /
Box Step-Ups	/ /	/ /	/ /	/ /
Dips	/ /	/ /	/ /	/ /
Squats	/ /	/ /	/ /	/ /
Pull-Ups*	/ /	/ /	/ /	/ /
Wall-Facing Squats	/ /	/ /	/ /	/ /
Isometric Hangs*	/ /	/ /	/ /	/ /

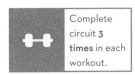 Complete circuit **3 times** in each workout.

P 207–221

* Starred exercises are for climbers with technical climbing objectives.

WEEKLY WORKOUT NOTES

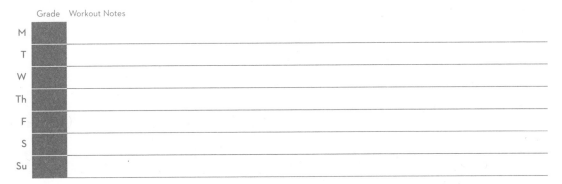

	Grade	Workout Notes
M		
T		
W		
Th		
F		
S		
Su		

TRANSITION PERIOD

DATE ＿＿ / ＿＿ / ＿＿ to ＿＿ / ＿＿ / ＿＿

> **!** This week's aerobic training volume should be only 5% more than what you completed in week 5. By now you should have a solid routine of **twice weekly** general and core strength training.

 P 183-221

WEEKLY TRAINING LOG

Activity by Time	Climb	Approach	Run	＿＿	＿＿	Altitude +/-	Time in Rec/Z 1	Time in Z 2	Time in Z 3	Time for Strength
M Plan										
Completed										
T Plan										
Completed										
W Plan										
Completed										
Th Plan										
Completed										
F Plan										
Completed										
S Plan										
Completed										
Su Plan										
Completed										

Target Hours This Week	
Actual Hours This Week	
Cumulative Training Hours	

During this week try to climb a minimum of 6-8 pitches that are 1-2 number grades below your current redpoint ability. Remember the principle of gradualness; resist the temptation to increase time spent climbing by more than 5-10% per week.

CLIMBING NOTES

Date	＿/＿/＿				＿/＿/＿				＿/＿/＿			
Vertical Gain												
Grades												
# of Pitches												

STRENGTH TRAINING

Core Routine	_/_/_		_/_/_	
Exercise	Reps	Weight	Reps	Weight
Strict Sit-Ups	/	/	/	/
Bird Dogs	/	/	/	/
Windshield Wipers	/	/	/	/
3-P/2-Point Planks	/	/	/	/
Kayakers	/	/	/	/

Core Routine				
Exercise	Reps	Weight	Reps	Weight
Super Push-Ups	/	/	/	/
Hanging Leg Raises	/	/	/	/
Bridges	/	/	/	/
Gymnast L-Sits	/	/	/	/
Side Planks	/	/	/	/

 Do this routine **twice** through with 30 seconds between exercises.

 P 192–206

General Strength Routine	_/_/_		_/_/_	
Exercise	Reps	Weight	Reps	Weight
TGUs	/ /	/ /	/ /	/ /
Split Squats	/ /	/ /	/ /	/ /
Push-Ups	/ /	/ /	/ /	/ /
Box Step-Ups	/ /	/ /	/ /	/ /
Dips	/ /	/ /	/ /	/ /
Squats	/ /	/ /	/ /	/ /
Pull-Ups*	/ /	/ /	/ /	/ /
Wall-Facing Squats	/ /	/ /	/ /	/ /
Isometric Hangs*	/ /	/ /	/ /	/ /

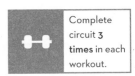 Complete circuit **3 times** in each workout.

 P 207–221

* Starred exercises are for climbers with technical climbing objectives.

WEEKLY WORKOUT NOTES

	Grade	Workout Notes
M		
T		
W		
Th		
F		
S		
Su		

DATE _____/_____/_____ to _____/_____/_____

> ❗ This week's aerobic training volume will again be approximately 5% more than what you completed in week 6. Keep pushing the strength training.
>
> 📖 P 183–221

WEEKLY TRAINING LOG

Activity by Time	Climb	Approach	Run	___	___	Altitude +/-	Time in Rec/Z 1	Time in Z 2	Time in Z 3	Time for Strength
M Plan										
Completed										
T Plan										
Completed										
W Plan										
Completed										
Th Plan										
Completed										
F Plan										
Completed										
S Plan										
Completed										
Su Plan										
Completed										

Target Hours This Week	
Actual Hours This Week	
Cumulative Training Hours	

> 🧗 During this week try to climb a minimum of 6–8 pitches that are 1–2 number grades below your current redpoint ability. Remember the principle of gradualness; resist the temptation to increase time spent climbing by more than 5–10% per week.

CLIMBING NOTES

Date	__/__/__	__/__/__	__/__/__
Vertical Gain			
Grades			
# of Pitches			

STRENGTH TRAINING

Core Routine	_/_/_		_/_/_	
Exercise	Reps	Weight	Reps	Weight
Strict Sit-Ups	/	/	/	/
Bird Dogs	/	/	/	/
Windshield Wipers	/	/	/	/
3-P/2-Point Planks	/	/	/	/
Kayakers	/	/	/	/

Core Routine				
Exercise	Reps	Weight	Reps	Weight
Super Push-Ups	/	/	/	/
Hanging Leg Raises	/	/	/	/
Bridges	/	/	/	/
Gymnast L-Sits	/	/	/	/
Side Planks	/	/	/	/

 Do this routine **twice** through with 30 seconds between exercises. P 192–206

General Strength Routine	_/_/_		_/_/_	
Exercise	Reps	Weight	Reps	Weight
TGUs	/ /	/ /	/ /	/ /
Split Squats	/ /	/ /	/ /	/ /
Push-Ups	/ /	/ /	/ /	/ /
Box Step-Ups	/ /	/ /	/ /	/ /
Dips	/ /	/ /	/ /	/ /
Squats	/ /	/ /	/ /	/ /
Pull-Ups*	/ /	/ /	/ /	/ /
Wall-Facing Squats	/ /	/ /	/ /	/ /
Isometric Hangs*	/ /	/ /	/ /	/ /

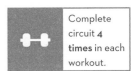 Complete circuit **4 times** in each workout. P 207–221

* Starred exercises are for climbers with technical climbing objectives.

WEEKLY WORKOUT NOTES

	Grade	Workout Notes
M		
T		
W		
Th		
F		
S		
Su		

TRANSITION PERIOD

DATE _____ / _____ / _____ to _____ / _____ / _____

! Consolidation week. This is an easy week to let your body consolidate the gains of the past 7 weeks of training. Your aerobic training and strength training volume should be approximately 50% of what you completed in week 7.

 P 183–221

WEEKLY TRAINING LOG

Activity by Time		Climb	Approach	Run	_____	_____	Altitude +/-	Time in Rec/Z 1	Time in Z 2	Time in Z 3	Time for Strength
M	Plan										
	Completed										
T	Plan										
	Completed										
W	Plan										
	Completed										
Th	Plan										
	Completed										
F	Plan										
	Completed										
S	Plan										
	Completed										
Su	Plan										
	Completed										

Target Hours This Week	
Actual Hours This Week	
Cumulative Training Hours	

 Climb no more than one day this week as rest and recovery is your goal. Aim for five pitches at least a full number grade below your redpoint ability. Err on the side of caution if you feel fatigued.

CLIMBING NOTES

Date	__/__/__	__/__/__	__/__/__
Vertical Gain			
Grades			
# of Pitches			

STRENGTH TRAINING

Core Routine	_/_/_	
Exercise	Reps	Weight
Strict Sit-Ups	/	/
Bird Dogs	/	/
Windshield Wipers	/	/
3-P/2-Point Planks	/	/
Kayakers	/	/
Super Push-Ups	/	/
Hanging Leg Raises	/	/
Bridges	/	/
Gymnast L-Sits	/	/
Side Planks	/	/

General Strength Routine	_/_/_					
Exercise	Reps			Weight		
TGUs	/	/	/	/	/	/
Split Squats	/	/	/	/	/	/
Push-Ups	/	/	/	/	/	/
Box Step-Ups	/	/	/	/	/	/
Dips	/	/	/	/	/	/
Squats	/	/	/	/	/	/
Pull-Ups*	/	/	/	/	/	/
Wall-Facing Squats	/	/	/	/	/	/
Isometric Hangs*	/	/	/	/	/	/

* Starred exercises are for climbers with technical climbing objectives.

 Do this routine **twice** through with 30 seconds between exercises.

P 192–206

 Complete circuit **4 times**.

P 207–221

WEEKLY WORKOUT NOTES

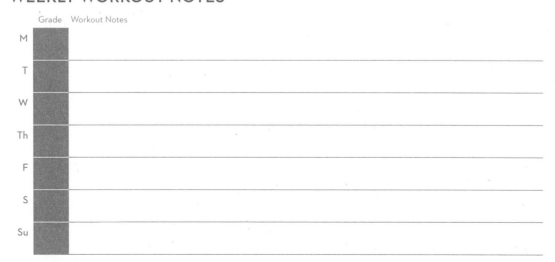

	Grade	Workout Notes
M		
T		
W		
Th		
F		
S		
Su		

BASE PERIOD PLANNING

Increasing your capacity for work

The Base Period is the time when you build your capacity for doing work. The more athletically mature you are, the more climbing specific this period can be. By the same token the less organized training background you have, the more this period should focus on building general fitness qualities. Many inexperienced athletes make the mistake of gravitating toward excess specificity in their base training. It is easy to be lured into the notion that there is a quick and easy route to the top of any sport by mimicking exactly what the pros do.

From your self-evaluation and the Transition Period you've just completed, you should have a good understanding of where you need extra work. During this period, all levels of climbers should focus on improving the weakest aspect of their set of alpine skills.

Since you can never have too much aerobic capacity for alpine climbing, that forms the cornerstone of all base training weeks. A twelve-week Base Period should be considered the minimum duration, and many people (especially those just starting out in training) will find a twenty-week Base Period to be very helpful in reaching a high level of physical preparation.

You'll get to be on a first-name basis with fatigue during the Base Period, so you'd better learn to be comfortable with it in all its nuanced forms. You need to learn to recognize good fatigue from bad. Only experience can teach you when more training will actually be better, and when enough is enough. Some fatigue is to be expected and even encouraged; this is the tiredness that you bounce back from after a good meal and a solid night's sleep. Other fatigue needs to be treated more carefully and incurred less frequently. In general, deep fatigue, stiffness, or soreness that lingers more than two days during normal training indicates that you've overreached. While overreaching can be a good stimulus from time to time when it is followed by appropriate recovery time, it should not be a constant in regular training.

Despite fatigue, you should occasionally feel noticeable improvements in your endurance. On these days you can tell that even while you are carrying some (and maybe even a lot of) fatigue, you are able to sustain a higher speed and/or power output than in previous weeks. Recognize this as both a sign of the training effect and especially as a time to back off, recover, and let the body adapt to this new level of fitness. Remember that the only way to expand your work capacity is to gently coax and nudge it forward.

In the final six or so weeks of the Base Period, it will become appropriate and beneficial to start inserting more climbing-specific workouts into the plan. These individual workouts should incorporate one, or at most two, aspects of the goal climb you are training for. Rely on the guiding principle of Gradualness. If you overreach in the Base Period it will upset the progression of training load you have so carefully planned. You'll need too much rest to recover from the overreach and may lose a week of what could have been valuable training time.

Follow these guidelines to build out your weekly plan:

- **One long Zone 1 workout** that comprises 25 to 30 percent of your total weekly volume on rolling, hilly terrain.

- **A hilly Zone 1–2 workout** that comprises 20 percent of your total weekly volume.

- **Make up the rest of the volume with Zone 1** or recovery aerobic work.

For technical climbing objectives add:

- **One day of technical alpine climbing**, or an approximation.

- **One day of cragging**, aiming for a large volume of climbing at about two grades below your onsight ability. Add or subtract climbing days as they are important relative to your goal.

- **If at any point you start to feel run down**, or detect the beginnings of illness, rest until you feel better.

- **Weeks 5 and 7** of this period will incorporate your first Zone 3 workouts.

PERIODIZING STRENGTH TRAINING FOR CLIMBERS

Chapters 4 & 5

For an in-depth review of strength training, study chapters 4 and 5 in *Training for the New Alpinism*. While the logbook will guide you with suggestions as your strength training progresses, it is best that you understand the material in the book before planning your own training.

A good plan follows this schedule:

- **General conditioning.** This prepares you for the heavy loads to come and is what you've been doing in the Transition Period. There are many variations of methods to use in this period. We explain one we have had good success with in our book. This period needs to be long for the beginner or for the athlete recovering from injury or from a long absence, and can be shortened for the advanced, healthy climber. If you skip this period you risk injury.

- **Max Strength.** This phase is for building a strength reserve—or stated another way, a high strength capacity—and can use semisport- to nonsport-specific exercises. These set and reps protocols are extremely well documented to be a simple way to build your strength capacity without adding weight or bulk to your body. Using the groups of strength exercises we recommend will help you to dramatically strengthen a wide range of muscles.

- **Muscular Endurance.** This converts the strength reserve into the specific strength requirements of alpine climbing by improving climbing-specific muscular endurance (ME). This builds on the strength phase and essentially trains your muscles to have a high strength capacity for longer.

Below are some considerations when tailoring both the Max Strength and Muscular Endurance training to best suit your aims.

- **In Max Strength training**, select exercises employing large muscle groups in a general or semisport-specific movement. Squats and box step-ups are two that address steep, uphill climbing movement in a general way with box step-ups being more specific as they are one-legged. Pull-ups, in their many variations, do the same thing for the upper body and will be as important as the lower-body strength exercises for the alpinist attempting difficult technical routes.

> Athletes don't strength train just for the sake of becoming stronger. They do so to enhance their athletic performance.

- **In Muscular Endurance workouts**, use the most sport-specific movements you can. The limitation we're concerned with in alpine climbing is normally going to be aerobic muscular endurance of the legs and hips over many hours. Similar training strategies have been in use for years with hard rock climbing. In that case the limitation is often going to be anaerobic endurance of the small forearm muscles for only a few seconds to several minutes. These two climbing goals need very different training stimuli. To develop both of these systems to high levels can require years' worth of delicately balancing the aerobic and anaerobic training loads. That is why climbing 5.12 at high altitudes is only within the reach of the most dedicated climbers.

Don't be afraid to change or progress exercises as you move through the General Conditioning, Max Strength, and Muscular Endurance training. There is no harm in sticking with one step-up exercise like box step-ups for the full eight-week Max Strength Period as it will allow you a good metric to gauge progress and it keeps things simple. However, it can be useful for more advanced climbers to progress from squats, to dead lifts, to box step-ups, to hill-sprints. Similarly in building upper-body Max Strength you can move from weighted pull-ups, to Frenchies, to typewriters, to front levers. This method adds variety to prevent boredom and staleness, and reaches slightly different muscle groups, giving a well-rounded training effect. Consider this second method mainly for advanced climbers with several years of strength training under their belts.

TRAINING BY CLIMBING

Chapter 14

In chapter 14 of *Training for the New Alpinism* we discuss a methodology for those more inclined to rely solely on climbing for their training. We do this not because it is the best approach to use, but more as an acknowledgement that many climbers will gravitate to this approach. For some this may in fact be a very successful way to train—especially if your basic fitness is already at a decent level but your climbing skills are relatively modest in terms of your goal climb. In that chapter we explain the methodology that adheres closely to correct training principles—using this approach is not an excuse to "just go climbing."

BASE PERIOD

DATE _____ / _____ / _____ to _____ / _____ / _____

> **!** This week's training volume should be approximately 10% higher than the highest training volume you actually completed during the Transition Period.

P 223-253

WEEKLY TRAINING LOG

Activity by Time		Climb	Approach	Run	____	____	Altitude + / -	Time in Rec/Z 1	Time in Z 2	Time in Z 3	Time for Strength
M	Plan										
	Completed										
T	Plan										
	Completed										
W	Plan										
	Completed										
Th	Plan										
	Completed										
F	Plan										
	Completed										
S	Plan										
	Completed										
Su	Plan										
	Completed										

Target Hours This Week	
Actual Hours This Week	
Cumulative Training Hours	

> Aim to complete 1 day of cragging. More cragging days may affect your ability to train your aerobic fitness level. If your absolute technical level needs to be increased for you to reach your goals, you may increase this to as many as 3 days of cragging. If your technical climbing ability is not the limiting factor, 1 day a week should be enough to keep your technique sharp.

CLIMBING NOTES

Date	_ / _ / _	_ / _ / _	_ / _ / _
Vertical Gain			
Grades			
# of Pitches			

STRENGTH TRAINING

Core Routine	__/__/__		__/__/__	
Exercise	Reps	Weight	Reps	Weight
Strict Sit-Ups				
Bird Dogs				
Windshield Wipers				
3-P/2-Point Planks				
Kayakers				

Core Routine				
Exercise	Reps	Weight	Reps	Weight
Super Push-Ups				
Hanging Leg Raises				
Bridges				
Gymnast L-Sits				
Side Planks				

 Do this routine **once** through as your warm-up.

 P 241–248

Max Strength Routine	__/__/__		__/__/__	
Exercise	Reps	Weight	Reps	Weight
	/ /	/ /	/ /	/ /
	/ /	/ /	/ /	/ /
	/ /	/ /	/ /	/ /
	/ /	/ /	/ /	/ /

 Complete 3–5 reps. Rest 3–5 minutes between sets. Do 3 sets.

 P 226–227

WEEKLY WORKOUT NOTES

	Grade	Workout Notes
M		
T		
W		
Th		
F		
S		
Su		

BASE

BASE PERIOD

DATE _____ / _____ / _____ to _____ / _____ / _____

> **!** This week's training volume should increase approximately 10-20% over last week. This is the biggest jump in volume so far and marks the beginning of a difficult couple of weeks of training.

P 223-253

WEEKLY TRAINING LOG

Activity by Time	Climb	Approach	Run	____	____	Altitude +/-	Time in Rec/Z 1	Time in Z 2	Time in Z 3	Time for Strength
M Plan										
Completed										
T Plan										
Completed										
W Plan										
Completed										
Th Plan										
Completed										
F Plan										
Completed										
S Plan										
Completed										
Su Plan										
Completed										

Target Hours This Week

Actual Hours This Week

Cumulative Training Hours

Aim to complete 1 day of cragging. More cragging days may affect your ability to train your aerobic fitness level. If your absolute technical level needs to be increased for you to reach your goals, you may increase this to as many as 3 days of cragging. If your technical climbing ability is not the limiting factor, 1 day a week should be enough to keep your technique sharp.

CLIMBING NOTES

Date	__/__/__	__/__/__	__/__/__
Vertical Gain			
Grades			
# of Pitches			

STRENGTH TRAINING

Core Routine	__/__/__		__/__/__	
Exercise	Reps	Weight	Reps	Weight
Strict Sit-Ups				
Bird Dogs				
Windshield Wipers				
3-P/2-Point Planks				
Kayakers				

Core Routine				
Exercise	Reps	Weight	Reps	Weight
Super Push-Ups				
Hanging Leg Raises				
Bridges				
Gymnast L-Sits				
Side Planks				

 Do this routine **once** through as your warm-up. P 241–248

Max Strength Routine	__/__/__		__/__/__	
Exercise	Reps	Weight	Reps	Weight
	/ /	/ /	/ /	/ /
	/ /	/ /	/ /	/ /
	/ /	/ /	/ /	/ /
	/ /	/ /	/ /	/ /

 Complete 3–5 reps. Rest 3–5 minutes between sets. Do 3 sets. P 226–227

WEEKLY WORKOUT NOTES

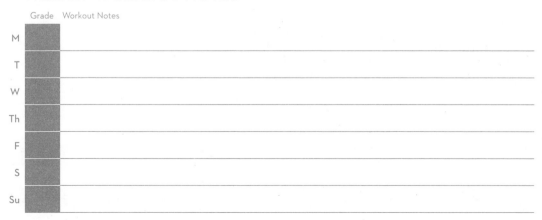

	Grade	Workout Notes
M		
T		
W		
Th		
F		
S		
Su		

BASE

BASE PERIOD

DATE _____/_____/_____ to _____/_____/_____

 ! This week's training volume should increase approximately 10-20% over last week. This week is probably going to be the most difficult week of training yet. Plan accordingly.

 P 223–253

WEEKLY TRAINING LOG

Activity by Time	Climb	Approach	Run	____	____	Altitude +/-	Time in Rec/Z 1	Time in Z 2	Time in Z 3	Time for Strength
M Plan										
Completed										
T Plan										
Completed										
W Plan										
Completed										
Th Plan										
Completed										
F Plan										
Completed										
S Plan										
Completed										
Su Plan										
Completed										

Target Hours This Week

Actual Hours This Week

Cumulative Training Hours

 Aim to complete 1 day of cragging. More cragging days may affect your ability to train your aerobic fitness level. If your absolute technical level needs to be increased for you to reach your goals, you may increase this to as many as 3 days of cragging. If your technical climbing ability is not the limiting factor, 1 day a week should be enough to keep your technique sharp.

CLIMBING NOTES

Date	_/_/_					_/_/_					_/_/_				
Vertical Gain															
Grades															
# of Pitches															

STRENGTH TRAINING

Core Routine	_/_/_		_/_/_	
Exercise	Reps	Weight	Reps	Weight
Strict Sit-Ups				
Bird Dogs				
Windshield Wipers				
3-P/2-Point Planks				
Kayakers				

Core Routine				
Exercise	Reps	Weight	Reps	Weight
Super Push-Ups				
Hanging Leg Raises				
Bridges				
Gymnast L-Sits				
Side Planks				

 Do this routine **once** through as your warm-up.   P 241–248

Max Strength Routine	_/_/_		_/_/_	
Exercise	Reps	Weight	Reps	Weight
	/ / /	/ / /	/ / /	/ / /
	/ / /	/ / /	/ / /	/ / /
	/ / /	/ / /	/ / /	/ / /
	/ / /	/ / /	/ / /	/ / /

 Complete 3–5 reps. Rest 3–5 minutes between sets. Do 4 sets.   P 226–227

WEEKLY WORKOUT NOTES

	Grade	Workout Notes
M		
T		
W		
Th		
F		
S		
Su		

BASE PERIOD

DATE ____/____/____ to ____/____/____

> **!** Reduce total training volume 25–35% from last week. This is a recovery week to allow you to absorb the previous training. The only thing that progresses this week is your strength training.

 P 223–253

WEEKLY TRAINING LOG

Activity by Time		Climb	Approach	Run	___	___	Altitude +/-	Time in Rec/Z 1	Time in Z 2	Time in Z 3	Time for Strength
M	Plan										
	Completed										
T	Plan										
	Completed										
W	Plan										
	Completed										
Th	Plan										
	Completed										
F	Plan										
	Completed										
S	Plan										
	Completed										
Su	Plan										
	Completed										

Target Hours This Week	
Actual Hours This Week	
Cumulative Training Hours	

 Aim to complete 1 day of cragging. More cragging days may affect your ability to train your aerobic fitness level. If your absolute technical level needs to be increased for you to reach your goals, you may increase this to as many as 3 days of cragging. If your technical climbing ability is not the limiting factor, 1 day a week should be enough to keep your technique sharp.

CLIMBING NOTES

Date	__/__/__				__/__/__				__/__/__			
Vertical Gain												
Grades												
# of Pitches												

STRENGTH TRAINING

Core Routine	__/__/__		__/__/__	
Exercise	Reps	Weight	Reps	Weight
Strict Sit-Ups				
Bird Dogs				
Windshield Wipers				
3-P/2-Point Planks				
Kayakers				

Core Routine				
Exercise	Reps	Weight	Reps	Weight
Super Push-Ups				
Hanging Leg Raises				
Bridges				
Gymnast L-Sits				
Side Planks				

 Do this routine **once** through as your warm-up. P 241–248

Max Strength Routine	__/__/__		__/__/__	
Exercise	Reps	Weight	Reps	Weight
	/ / /	/ / /	/ / /	/ / /
	/ / /	/ / /	/ / /	/ / /
	/ / /	/ / /	/ / /	/ / /
	/ / /	/ / /	/ / /	/ / /

 Complete 3–5 reps. Rest 3–5 minutes between sets. Do 4 sets. Increase weight when possible. P 226–227

WEEKLY WORKOUT NOTES

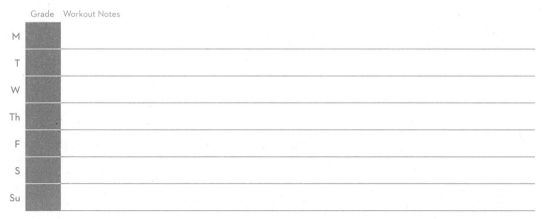

	Grade	Workout Notes
M		
T		
W		
Th		
F		
S		
Su		

BASE

BASE PERIOD

DATE _____ / _____ / _____ to _____ / _____ / _____

> **!** This week's training volume should equal Base Period week 3's completed training volume. This is another hard week, and you will have your first Zone 3 workout, which should make up 20% of this week's volume.

P 223–253

WEEKLY TRAINING LOG

Activity by Time	Climb	Approach	Run	___	___	Altitude +/-	Time in Rec/Z 1	Time in Z 2	Time in Z 3	Time for Strength
M Plan										
Completed										
T Plan										
Completed										
W Plan										
Completed										
Th Plan										
Completed										
F Plan										
Completed										
S Plan										
Completed										
Su Plan										
Completed										

Target Hours This Week	
Actual Hours This Week	
Cumulative Training Hours	

> Aim to complete 1 day of cragging. More cragging days may affect your ability to train your aerobic fitness level. If your absolute technical level needs to be increased for you to reach your goals, you may increase this to as many as 3 days of cragging. If your technical climbing ability is not the limiting factor, 1 day a week should be enough to keep your technique sharp.

CLIMBING NOTES

Date	_/_/_	_/_/_	_/_/_
Vertical Gain			
Grades			
# of Pitches			

STRENGTH TRAINING

Core Routine	__/__/__		__/__/__	
Exercise	Reps	Weight	Reps	Weight
Strict Sit-Ups				
Bird Dogs				
Windshield Wipers				
3-P/2-Point Planks				
Kayakers				

Core Routine				
Exercise	Reps	Weight	Reps	Weight
Super Push-Ups				
Hanging Leg Raises				
Bridges				
Gymnast L-Sits				
Side Planks				

 Do this routine **once** through as your warm-up.

 P 241-248

Max Strength Routine	__/__/__		__/__/__	
Exercise	Reps	Weight	Reps	Weight
	/ / / /	/ / / /	/ / / /	/ / / /
	/ / / /	/ / / /	/ / / /	/ / / /
	/ / / /	/ / / /	/ / / /	/ / / /
	/ / / /	/ / / /	/ / / /	/ / / /

 Complete 3–5 reps. Rest 3–5 minutes between sets. Do 5 sets.

 P 226-227

WEEKLY WORKOUT NOTES

	Grade	Workout Notes
M		
T		
W		
Th		
F		
S		
Su		

BASE

BASE PERIOD

DATE _____ / _____ / _____ to _____ / _____ / _____

> **!** This week's training is the same as week 5 to allow ideal training adaptation.

 P 223-253

WEEKLY TRAINING LOG

Activity by Time		Climb	Approach	Run	____	____	Altitude +/-	Time in Rec/Z 1	Time in Z 2	Time in Z 3	Time for Strength
M	Plan										
	Completed										
T	Plan										
	Completed										
W	Plan										
	Completed										
Th	Plan										
	Completed										
F	Plan										
	Completed										
S	Plan										
	Completed										
Su	Plan										
	Completed										

Target Hours This Week

Actual Hours This Week

Cumulative Training Hours

 Aim to complete 1 day of cragging. More cragging days may affect your ability to train your aerobic fitness level. If your absolute technical level needs to be increased for you to reach your goals, you may increase this to as many as 3 days of cragging. If your technical climbing ability is not the limiting factor, 1 day a week should be enough to keep your technique sharp.

CLIMBING NOTES

Date	__/__/__							__/__/__							__/__/__						
Vertical Gain																					
Grades																					
# of Pitches																					

STRENGTH TRAINING

Core Routine	__/__/__		__/__/__	
Exercise	Reps	Weight	Reps	Weight
Strict Sit-Ups				
Bird Dogs				
Windshield Wipers				
3-P/2-Point Planks				
Kayakers				

Core Routine				
Exercise	Reps	Weight	Reps	Weight
Super Push-Ups		·		
Hanging Leg Raises				
Bridges				
Gymnast L-Sits				
Side Planks				

 Do this routine **once** through as your warm-up. P 241-248

Max Strength Routine	__/__/__		__/__/__	
Exercise	Reps	Weight	Reps	Weight
	/ / / /	/ / / /	/ / / /	/ / / /
	/ / / /	/ / / /	/ / / /	/ / / /
	/ / / /	/ / / /	/ / / /	/ / / /
	/ / / /	/ / / /	/ / / /	/ / / /

 Complete 3–5 reps. Rest 3–5 minutes between sets. Do 5 sets. P 226-227

WEEKLY WORKOUT NOTES

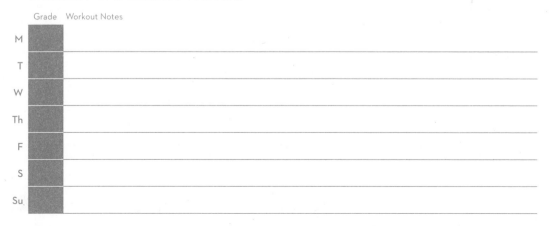

	Grade	Workout Notes
M		
T		
W		
Th		
F		
S		
Su		

BASE PERIOD

DATE _____/_____/_____ **to** _____/_____/_____

> **!** This week's training volume should increase by 25% over last week's completed training volume. You will conduct one Zone 3 workout that takes about half as long as the Zone 3 workout you completed two weeks ago. From here on out cap your strength training time at three hours per week.
>
> P 223–253

WEEKLY TRAINING LOG

Activity by Time		Climb	Approach	Run	___	___	Altitude +/-	Time in Rec/Z 1	Time in Z 2	Time in Z 3	Time for Strength
M	Plan										
	Completed										
T	Plan										
	Completed										
W	Plan										
	Completed										
Th	Plan										
	Completed										
F	Plan										
	Completed										
S	Plan										
	Completed										
Su	Plan										
	Completed										

Target Hours This Week	
Actual Hours This Week	
Cumulative Training Hours	

> Aim to complete 1 day of cragging. More cragging days may affect your ability to train your aerobic fitness level. If your absolute technical level needs to be increased for you to reach your goals, you may increase this to as many as 3 days of cragging. If your technical climbing ability is not the limiting factor, 1 day a week should be enough to keep your technique sharp.

CLIMBING NOTES

Date	__/__/__						__/__/__						__/__/__				
Vertical Gain																	
Grades																	
# of Pitches																	

STRENGTH TRAINING

Core Routine	_ / _ / _		_ / _ / _	
Exercise	Reps	Weight	Reps	Weight
Strict Sit-Ups				
Bird Dogs				
Windshield Wipers				
3-P/2-Point Planks				
Kayakers				

Core Routine				
Exercise	Reps	Weight	Reps	Weight
Super Push-Ups				
Hanging Leg Raises				
Bridges				
Gymnast L-Sits				
Side Planks				

 Do this routine **once** through as your warm-up.

 P 241-248

Max Strength Routine	_ / _ / _		_ / _ / _	
Exercise	Reps	Weight	Reps	Weight
	/ / / / /	/ / / / /	/ / / / /	/ / / / /
	/ / / / /	/ / / / /	/ / / / /	/ / / / /
	/ / / / /	/ / / / /	/ / / / /	/ / / / /
	/ / / / /	/ / / / /	/ / / / /	/ / / / /

 Complete 3–5 reps. Rest 3–5 minutes between sets. Do 6 sets. Increase weight when possible.

 P 226-227

WEEKLY WORKOUT NOTES

	Grade	Workout Notes
M		
T		
W		
Th		
F		
S		
Su		

BASE

BASE PERIOD

DATE ____/____/____ to ____/____/____

> **!** This week's training volume should decrease by 50% from last week's completed training volume. This is an important rest week before launching into the next cycle of base training.
>
> 📖 P 223–253

WEEKLY TRAINING LOG

Activity by Time		Climb	Approach	Run	___	___	Altitude +/-	Time in Rec/Z 1	Time in Z 2	Time in Z 3	Time for Strength
M	Plan										
	Completed										
T	Plan										
	Completed										
W	Plan										
	Completed										
Th	Plan										
	Completed										
F	Plan										
	Completed										
S	Plan										
	Completed										
Su	Plan										
	Completed										

Target Hours This Week	
Actual Hours This Week	
Cumulative Training Hours	

 Aim to complete 1 day of cragging. More cragging days may affect your ability to train your aerobic fitness level. If your absolute technical level needs to be increased for you to reach your goals, you may increase this to as many as 3 days of cragging. If your technical climbing ability is not the limiting factor, 1 day a week should be enough to keep your technique sharp.

CLIMBING NOTES

Date	__/__/__			__/__/__			__/__/__		
Vertical Gain									
Grades									
# of Pitches									

STRENGTH TRAINING

Core Routine	__/__/__		__/__/__	
Exercise	Reps	Weight	Reps	Weight
Strict Sit-Ups				
Bird Dogs				
Windshield Wipers				
3-P/2-Point Planks				
Kayakers				

Core Routine				
Exercise	Reps	Weight	Reps	Weight
Super Push-Ups				
Hanging Leg Raises				
Bridges				
Gymnast L-Sits				
Side Planks				

 Do this routine **once** through as your warm-up. P 241-248

Max Strength Routine	__/__/__		__/__/__	
Exercise	Reps	Weight	Reps	Weight
	/ / / / /	/ / / / /	/ / / / /	/ / / / /
	/ / / / /	/ / / / /	/ / / / /	/ / / / /
	/ / / / /	/ / / / /	/ / / / /	/ / / / /
	/ / / / /	/ / / / /	/ / / / /	/ / / / /

 Complete 3–5 reps. Rest 3–5 minutes between sets. Do 6 sets. Increase weight when possible. P 226-227

WEEKLY WORKOUT NOTES

	Grade	Workout Notes
M		
T		
W		
Th		
F		
S		
Su		

NOTES FOR WEEKS 9–16

Now begins the conversion to the sport-specificity component of your training, with the aim being to dramatically improve muscular endurance (ME) over the next eight weeks. This is where the training for a technical versus nontechnical climb will begin to diverge, and it will be necessary to carefully reread pages 249–253 to understand the special requirements needed to prepare for technical climbs. Do these Muscular Endurance workouts once or twice a week with a progression in difficulty from week to week as outlined in the log pages. The following pages are templates for nontechnical mountaineering objectives, and we have left it up to readers to add the technical components that best match their objective by using the guidelines laid out in *Training for the New Alpinism*.

P 249-253

Please see pages 233–241 in *Training for the New Alpinism* for a review of Muscular Endurance training.

P 233-241

The core routine and Max Strength workouts will drop to maintenance levels by doing abbreviated versions of your previous core and Max Strength workouts once every seven to ten days. These workouts are done by choosing three or four of your most challenging core exercises and doing those to failure a couple of times. This will be enough to maintain good core strength. Do the same with the Max Strength exercises. Pick a couple of favorites and do two or three sets of two or three reps.

These short maintenance workouts should feel fun, easy, and leave you feeling energized.

From here on out the Base Period Muscular Endurance (ME) training will make up a significant portion of your training. Regardless of whether you are carrying water jugs up a hill, doing laps in the climbing gym, or hand walking on a treadmill, it is very demanding work and all of what you have done up to this point has been to prepare you for this. Make the most of it and you'll reap huge gains. Overdo it and you could be reduced to an overtrained, quivering mess. In our experience with these workouts we have found that very fit individuals who have a strong aerobic and strength base can handle two ME workouts in a week at the most and make gains. More than twice per week is too taxing even for the most developed athletes.

Start with one session per week for the first three weeks until you get a handle on the workouts. By the fourteenth week of the Base Period, you can begin to experiment with fitting two lower-body ME workouts into the week if you feel up to it. If you are planning a nontechnical route, focus on the uphill water carries for both of the ME sessions. If your goal is a route with lots of belayed climbing, then mix in sessions that include upper-body ME workouts. An appropriate workout for a technical climber could also be done on the rock or ice by employing the same principle of progression in loading from workout to workout. Your goal is to gradually build your volume of training in this hard effort zone. Many laps at sub-max grade with short to no rest will be better than fewer laps at a higher intensity that require longer rests. It will require some experimentation for you to decide the best mix of upper- and lower-body ME workouts so that you feel you get the work where you need it the most.

Since even technically difficult climbs still require most of your locomotion coming from the legs, we recommend biasing this training toward the hill climbs with water jugs.

Continue to follow these guidelines to build out your weekly plan:

- **One long Zone 1 workout** that comprises 25 to 30 percent of your total weekly volume on rolling, hilly terrain.

- **A hilly Zone 1–2 workout** that comprises 20 percent of your total weekly volume.

- **Make up the rest of the volume** with Zone 1 or recovery aerobic work.

For technical climbing objectives add:

- **One day of technical alpine climbing**, or an approximation.

- **One day of cragging**, aiming for a large volume of climbing at about two grades below your onsight ability. Add or subtract climbing days as they are important relative to your goal.

Hint: You should feel a gain in strength and endurance from workout to workout. If you do not, then you need to space them further apart with more easy workouts to ensure enough recovery before you tackle the next one.

- **If at any point you start to feel run down**, or detect the beginnings of illness, rest until you feel better.

In week 9 you should plan two long Zone 1 workouts that comprise 20 percent and 30 percent of your total weekly volume, respectively, and an uphill-focused Zone 3 workout that comprises 10 percent of your weekly volume. During week 9 is also the time to start carrying weight during your Zone 1 workouts. Start with 10 percent of your body weight. At this point it's okay to combine two Zone 1 workouts into one long day out.

NOTES ON CLIMBING FOR WEEKS 9–16

Aim to complete one day of cragging. More cragging days will likely affect your ability to train your aerobic fitness and muscular endurance. When you do climb, go until you feel yourself fatiguing to the point that you're making errors in technique. Once that happens, you're done. If you don't think your technical climbing ability is the limiting factor, one day a week will be enough to keep your technique sharp.

If your absolute technical climbing ability needs to be increased for you to reach your goals you may increase the number of cragging days to as many as three days per week. If this is your situation we recommend that you replace the Muscular Endurance workouts with these additional cragging days.

BASE PERIOD

DATE _____ / _____ / _____ to _____ / _____ / _____

! This week's training volume should be approximately the same as Base Period week 7's volume. This week you'll start to incorporate taxing Muscular Endurance workouts, so reduce the Max Strength and core routines to maintenance levels as discussed.

P 223–253

WEEKLY TRAINING LOG

Activity by Time		Climb	Approach	Run	_____	_____	Altitude + / -	Time in Rec/Z 1	Time in Z 2	Time in Z 3	Time for Strength
M	Plan										
	Completed										
T	Plan										
	Completed										
W	Plan										
	Completed										
Th	Plan										
	Completed										
F	Plan										
	Completed										
S	Plan										
	Completed										
Su	Plan										
	Completed										

Target Hours This Week	
Actual Hours This Week	
Cumulative Training Hours	

Resist the temptation to increase the time spent climbing by more than 5–10% per week. When you climb alpine routes, record total time and the grade of the most difficult pitch.

CLIMBING NOTES

Date	_ / _ / _					_ / _ / _					_ / _ / _				
Vertical Gain															
Grades															
# of Pitches															

STRENGTH TRAINING

Core Routine	_ / _ / _	
Exercise	Reps	Weight

Starting this week do a simplified core routine only **once** and as a warm-up for your simplified Max Strength workout. Choose your four most challenging core exercises.

P 249–251

Max Strength Routine	_ / _ / _	
Exercise	Reps	Weight
	/ /	/ /
	/ /	/ /
	/ /	/ /
	/ /	/ /

Muscular Endurance	_ / _ / _	
	Lower Body	Upper Body
Distance		
Elevation +/-		
Time		
Weight		

Complete 2-3 reps. Rest 3-5 minutes between sets. Do 2-3 sets. Increase weight when possible.

Beginning this week we introduce one Muscular Endurance workout per week. The upper-body component is required only if you are pursuing technical climbing objectives.

P 233–241

WEEKLY WORKOUT NOTES

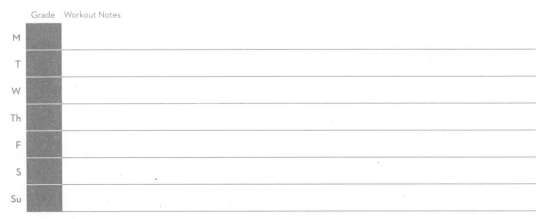

	Grade	Workout Notes
M		
T		
W		
Th		
F		
S		
Su		

BASE

BASE PERIOD

DATE ____ / ____ / ____ to ____ / ____ / ____

> **!** This week's training volume should increase 5-10% over last week's volume. Try to get off trail to practice moving efficiently over rough, mountainous terrain.
>
> 📖 P 223-253

WEEKLY TRAINING LOG

Activity by Time	Climb	Approach	Run	____	____	Altitude +/-	Time in Rec/Z 1	Time in Z 2	Time in Z 3	Time for Strength
M Plan										
Completed										
T Plan										
Completed										
W Plan										
Completed										
Th Plan										
Completed										
F Plan										
Completed										
S Plan										
Completed										
Su Plan										
Completed										

Target Hours This Week

Actual Hours This Week

Cumulative Training Hours

> Resist the temptation to increase the time spent climbing by more than 5-10% per week. When you climb alpine routes, record total time and the grade of the most difficult pitch.

CLIMBING NOTES

Date ___/___/___   ___/___/___   ___/___/___

Vertical Gain															
Grades															
# of Pitches															

STRENGTH TRAINING

Core Routine	__/__/__	
Exercise	Reps	Weight

Do a simplified core routine only **once** as a warm-up for your simplified Max Strength workout. Choose your four most challenging core exercises.

P 249–251

Max Strength Routine	__/__/__	
Exercise	Reps	Weight
	/ /	/ /
	/ /	/ /
	/ /	/ /
	/ /	/ /

Muscular Endurance	__/__/__	
	Lower Body	Upper Body
Distance		
Elevation +/-		
Time		
Weight		

P 233–241

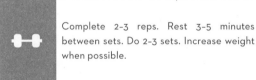

Complete 2–3 reps. Rest 3–5 minutes between sets. Do 2–3 sets. Increase weight when possible.

WEEKLY WORKOUT NOTES

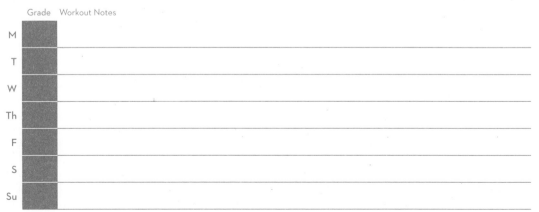

	Grade	Workout Notes
M		
T		
W		
Th		
F		
S		
Su		

BASE PERIOD

DATE _____ / _____ / _____ to _____ / _____ / _____

> **!** This week's training volume should again increase 5–10% over last week's volume. This is a very demanding week, but next week is a rest week. Hang in there!

P 223–253

WEEKLY TRAINING LOG

Activity by Time		Climb	Approach	Run	___	___	Altitude +/-	Time in Rec/Z 1	Time in Z 2	Time in Z 3	Time for Strength
M	Plan										
	Completed										
T	Plan										
	Completed										
W	Plan										
	Completed										
Th	Plan										
	Completed										
F	Plan										
	Completed										
S	Plan										
	Completed										
Su	Plan										
	Completed										

Target Hours This Week	
Actual Hours This Week	
Cumulative Training Hours	

> Resist the temptation to increase the time spent climbing by more than 5–10% per week. When you climb alpine routes, record total time and the grade of the most difficult pitch.

CLIMBING NOTES

Date   __/__/__   __/__/__   __/__/__

Vertical Gain																		
Grades																		
# of Pitches																		

STRENGTH TRAINING

Core Routine	__/__/__	
Exercise	Reps	Weight

Do a simplified core routine only **once** as a warm-up for your simplified Max Strength workout. Choose your four most challenging core exercises.

P 249-251

Max Strength Routine	__/__/__	
Exercise	Reps	Weight
	/ /	/ /
	/ /	/ /
	/ /	/ /
	/ /	/ /

Complete 2-3 reps. Rest 3-5 minutes between sets. Do 2-3 sets. Increase weight when possible.

Muscular Endurance	__/__/__	
	Lower Body	Upper Body
Distance		
Elevation +/-		
Time		
Weight		

P 233-241

BASE

WEEKLY WORKOUT NOTES

	Grade	Workout Notes
M		
T		
W		
Th		
F		
S		
Su		

BASE PERIOD

DATE _____ / _____ / _____ to _____ / _____ / _____

> **!** Recovery week. Cut your training volume in half and do 90% of your volume in Zone 1, 10% of your volume in Zone 2. You are going to feel tired this week, concentrate on getting as much sleep as possible. Eat well.
>
> 📖 P 223–253

WEEKLY TRAINING LOG

Activity by Time	Climb	Approach	Run	____	____	Altitude +/-	Time in Rec/Z 1	Time in Z 2	Time in Z 3	Time for Strength
M Plan										
Completed										
T Plan										
Completed										
W Plan										
Completed										
Th Plan										
Completed										
F Plan										
Completed										
S Plan										
Completed										
Su Plan										
Completed										

Target Hours This Week	
Actual Hours This Week	
Cumulative Training Hours	

> Resist the temptation to increase the time spent climbing by more than 5–10% per week. When you climb alpine routes, record total time and the grade of the most difficult pitch.

CLIMBING NOTES

Date	__/__/__			__/__/__			__/__/__		
Vertical Gain									
Grades									
# of Pitches									

STRENGTH TRAINING

Core Routine	_ / _ / _	
Exercise	Reps	Weight

Do a simplified core routine only **once** as a warm-up for your simplified Max Strength workout. Choose your 4 most challenging core exercises.

P 249-251

Max Strength Routine	_ / _ / _	
Exercise	Reps	Weight
	/ /	/ /
	/ /	/ /
	/ /	/ /
	/ /	/ /

Muscular Endurance	_ / _ / _	
	Lower Body	Upper Body
Distance		
Elevation +/-		
Time		
Weight		

P 233-241

Complete 2-3 reps. Rest 3-5 minutes between sets. Do 2-3 sets. Increase weight when possible. Time spent strength training does not change this week.

WEEKLY WORKOUT NOTES

	Grade	Workout Notes
M		
T		
W		
Th		
F		
S		
Su		

BASE PERIOD

DATE _____ / _____ / _____ to _____ / _____ / _____

> **!** This week and the next week are consolidation weeks. Maintain week 11's training volume: 75% of volume in Zone 1, 10% of volume in Zone 3, 15% of your volume, or a maximum of 3 hours, should be strength training. If all is going according to plan, you will notice that you can now do the same work as you did in week 11, but with less fatigue.
>
> P 223–253

WEEKLY TRAINING LOG

Activity by Time		Climb	Approach	Run	____	____	Altitude +/-	Time in Rec/Z 1	Time in Z 2	Time in Z 3	Time for Strength
M	Plan										
	Completed										
T	Plan										
	Completed										
W	Plan										
	Completed										
Th	Plan										
	Completed										
F	Plan										
	Completed										
S	Plan										
	Completed										
Su	Plan										
	Completed										

Target Hours This Week

Actual Hours This Week

Cumulative Training Hours

> Resist the temptation to increase the time spent climbing by more than 5–10% per week. When you climb alpine routes, record total time and the grade of the most difficult pitch.

CLIMBING NOTES

Date _ / _ / _   _ / _ / _   _ / _ / _

Vertical Gain												
Grades												
# of Pitches												

STRENGTH TRAINING

Core Routine	__/__/__	
Exercise	Reps	Weight

Do a simplified core routine only **once** as a warm-up for your simplified Max Strength workout. Choose your 4 most challenging core exercises.

P 249-251

Max Strength Routine	__/__/__	
Exercise	Reps	Weight
	/ /	/ /
	/ /	/ /
	/ /	/ /
	/ /	/ /

Muscular Endurance	__/__/__	
	Lower Body	Upper Body
Distance		
Elevation +/-		
Time		
Weight		

P 233-241

Complete 2-3 reps. Rest 3-5 minutes between sets. Do 2-3 sets. Increase weight when possible.

WEEKLY WORKOUT NOTES

	Grade	Workout Notes
M		
T		
W		
Th		
F		
S		
Su		

BASE

BASE PERIOD

DATE ____ / ____ / ____ to ____ / ____ / ____

> **!** Same training volume as last week: 75% of volume in Zone 1, 10% of volume in Zone 3, 15% of your volume, or a maximum of 3 hours, should be strength training.
>
> P 223-253

WEEKLY TRAINING LOG

Activity by Time		Climb	Approach	Run	____	____	Altitude +/-	Time in Rec/Z 1	Time in Z 2	Time in Z 3	Time for Strength
M	Plan										
	Completed										
T	Plan										
	Completed										
W	Plan										
	Completed										
Th	Plan										
	Completed										
F	Plan										
	Completed										
S	Plan										
	Completed										
Su	Plan										
	Completed										

Target Hours This Week

Actual Hours This Week

Cumulative Training Hours

> Resist the temptation to increase the time spent climbing by more than 5–10% per week. When you climb alpine routes, record total time and the grade of the most difficult pitch.

CLIMBING NOTES

Date	__/__/__					__/__/__					__/__/__				
Vertical Gain															
Grades															
# of Pitches															

STRENGTH TRAINING

Core Routine	__ / __ / __	
Exercise	Reps	Weight

Max Strength Routine	__ / __ / __	
Exercise	Reps	Weight
	/ /	/ /
	/ /	/ /
	/ /	/ /
	/ /	/ /

 Continue doing a simplified core routine **once** as a warm-up for your simplified Max Strength workout.

 Complete 2-3 reps. Rest 3-5 minutes between sets. Do 2-3 sets. Increase weight when possible.

Muscular Endurance	__ / __ / __	
	Lower Body	Upper Body
Distance		
Elevation +/-		
Time		
Weight		

Muscular Endurance	__ / __ / __	
	Lower Body	Upper Body
Distance		
Elevation +/-		
Time		
Weight		

 P 233-241

 Starting this week you can begin to experiment with doing 2 Muscular Endurance workouts per week.

WEEKLY WORKOUT NOTES

	Grade	Workout Notes
M		
T		
W		
Th		
F		
S		
Su		

BASE PERIOD

DATE ____/____/____ to ____/____/____

> **!** This is a Volume Overload Week. Plan a 20% increase over week 14's training volume. You will be very tired this week. Pay very close attention to your recovery and stress level. We can't overemphasize how important recovery is right now. Don't get sick and sink the ship!
>
> P 223-253

WEEKLY TRAINING LOG

Activity by Time		Climb	Approach	Run	____	____	Altitude +/-	Time in Rec/Z 1	Time in Z 2	Time in Z 3	Time for Strength
M	Plan										
	Completed										
T	Plan										
	Completed										
W	Plan										
	Completed										
Th	Plan										
	Completed										
F	Plan										
	Completed										
S	Plan										
	Completed										
Su	Plan										
	Completed										

Target Hours This Week	
Actual Hours This Week	
Cumulative Training Hours	

> Resist the temptation to increase the time spent climbing by more than 5–10% per week. When you climb alpine routes, record total time and the grade of the most difficult pitch.

CLIMBING NOTES

Date	__/__/__	__/__/__	__/__/__
Vertical Gain			
Grades			
# of Pitches			

STRENGTH TRAINING

Core Routine	_ / _ / _	
Exercise	Reps	Weight

Max Strength Routine	_ / _ / _	
Exercise	Reps	Weight
	/ /	/ /
	/ /	/ /
	/ /	/ /
	/ /	/ /

 Continue doing a simplified core routine **once** as a warm-up for your simplified Max Strength workout.

 Complete 2–3 reps. Rest 3–5 minutes between sets. Do 2–3 sets. Increase weight when possible.

Muscular Endurance	_ / _ / _	
	Lower Body	Upper Body
Distance		
Elevation +/-		
Time		
Weight		

Muscular Endurance	_ / _ / _	
	Lower Body	Upper Body
Distance		
Elevation +/-		
Time		
Weight		

 P 233-241

 Continue to experiment with doing 2 Muscular Endurance workouts per week.

WEEKLY WORKOUT NOTES

	Grade	Workout Notes
M		
T		
W		
Th		
F		
S		
Su		

BASE PERIOD

DATE _____/_____/_____ to _____/_____/_____

| ! | Rest week. Whew! You've earned this week! Drop your training volume 50–70% from last week. Recovery, sleep, and nutrition are the name of the game now. Still, you have to plan 80% of your time in recovery or Zone 1, do a short Zone 3, and complete 2 maintenance-strength workouts. | 📖 P 223–253 |

WEEKLY TRAINING LOG

Activity by Time		Climb	Approach	Run	____	____	Altitude +/-	Time in Rec/Z 1	Time in Z 2	Time in Z 3	Time for Strength
M	Plan										
	Completed										
T	Plan										
	Completed										
W	Plan										
	Completed										
Th	Plan										
	Completed										
F	Plan										
	Completed										
S	Plan										
	Completed										
Su	Plan										
	Completed										

Target Hours This Week	
Actual Hours This Week	
Cumulative Training Hours	

Resist the temptation to increase the time spent climbing by more than 5–10% per week. When you climb alpine routes, record total time and the grade of the most difficult pitch.

CLIMBING NOTES

Date	__/__/__	__/__/__	__/__/__
Vertical Gain			
Grades			
# of Pitches			

STRENGTH TRAINING

Core Routine	_/_/_	
Exercise	Reps	Weight

Max Strength Routine	_/_/_	
Exercise	Reps	Weight
	/ /	/ /
	/ /	/ /
	/ /	/ /
	/ /	/ /

 Continue doing a simplified core routine **once** as a warm-up for your simplified Max Strength workout.

 Complete 2-3 reps. Rest 3-5 minutes between sets. Do 2-3 sets. Increase weight when possible.

Muscular Endurance	_/_/_	
	Lower Body	Upper Body
Distance		
Elevation +/-		
Time		
Weight		

Muscular Endurance	_/_/_	
	Lower Body	Upper Body
Distance		
Elevation +/-		
Time		
Weight		

P 233-241

 Continue to experiment with doing 2 Muscular Endurance workouts per week.

WEEKLY WORKOUT NOTES

	Grade	Workout Notes
M		
T		
W		
Th		
F		
S		
Su		

BASE

BASE PERIOD

DATE _____ / _____ / _____ to _____ / _____ / _____

> **!** Use week 15's volume. Complete two long Zone 1 workouts that are 30% and 20% of your weekly volume, respectively. All remaining volume is done at recovery or Zone 1 intensities. These are the weeks that will produce the most gains.
>
> P 223-253

WEEKLY TRAINING LOG

Activity by Time		Climb	Approach	Run	____	____	Altitude +/-	Time in Rec/Z 1	Time in Z 2	Time in Z 3	Time for Strength
M	Plan										
	Completed										
T	Plan										
	Completed										
W	Plan										
	Completed										
Th	Plan										
	Completed										
F	Plan										
	Completed										
S	Plan										
	Completed										
Su	Plan										
	Completed										

Target Hours This Week	
Actual Hours This Week	
Cumulative Training Hours	

 Drop cragging so that more time can be spent on Muscular Endurance training and alpine climbs.

CLIMBING NOTES

Date	_/_/_	_/_/_	_/_/_
Vertical Gain			
Grades			
# of Pitches			

STRENGTH TRAINING

Muscular Endurance	_ / _ / _	
	Lower Body	_____ Body
Distance		
Elevation +/-		
Time		
Weight		

Do 1 upper- and 1 lower-body Muscular Endurance workout if you are doing a technical climb, or do 2 Muscular Endurance lower-body workouts if you are doing a climb with low (for you) technical challenge. Make one of these a good one—try to exceed your previous efforts. No Max Strength or core workouts this week.

WEEKLY WORKOUT NOTES

	Grade	Workout Notes
M		
T		
W		
Th		
F		
S		
Su		

BASE

DATE _____ / _____ / _____ to _____ / _____ / _____

> **!** Drop this week's training volume by 25% from last week. Keep the two long workouts comprising approximately 30% and 20% of your weekly volume. Remaining volume is done at recovery intensity. This is an important consolidation week: rest well, eat well.
>
> P 223–253

WEEKLY TRAINING LOG

Activity by Time	Climb	Approach	Run	___	___	Altitude +/-	Time in Rec/Z 1	Time in Z 2	Time in Z 3	Time for Strength
M Plan										
Completed										
T Plan										
Completed										
W Plan										
Completed										
Th Plan										
Completed										
F Plan										
Completed										
S Plan										
Completed										
Su Plan										
Completed										

Target Hours This Week	
Actual Hours This Week	
Cumulative Training Hours	

> Drop cragging so that more time can be spent on Muscular Endurance training and alpine climbs.

CLIMBING NOTES

Date	__/__/__	__/__/__	__/__/__
Vertical Gain			
Grades			
# of Pitches			

STRENGTH TRAINING

Core Routine	_/_/_	
Exercise	Reps	Weight

Muscular Endurance	_/_/_	
	Lower Body	Upper Body
Distance		
Elevation +/-		
Time		
Weight		

 Do 1 complete Max Strength workout using the abbreviated core routine as your warm-up.

 On another day do 1 Muscular Endurance workout of your choice: upper or lower body.

Max Strength Routine	_/_/_	
Exercise	Reps	Weight
	/ / / / /	/ / / / /
	/ / / / /	/ / / / /
	/ / / / /	/ / / / /
	/ / / / /	/ / / / /

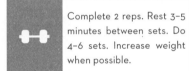 Complete 2 reps. Rest 3–5 minutes between sets. Do 4–6 sets. Increase weight when possible.

WEEKLY WORKOUT NOTES

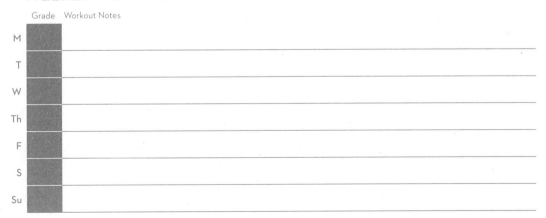

	Grade	Workout Notes
M		
T		
W		
Th		
F		
S		
Su		

BASE PERIOD

DATE _____ / _____ / _____ to _____ / _____ / _____

> **!** Use week 17's volume. Complete 2 long Zone 1 workouts that are 30% and 20% of your weekly volume, respectively. All remaining volume is done at recovery or Zone 1 intensities. Concentrate on preparing for and recovering from the strength workouts; these will be hugely beneficial at this stage.
>
> P 223–253

WEEKLY TRAINING LOG

Activity by Time	Climb	Approach	Run	___	___	Altitude +/-	Time in Rec/Z 1	Time in Z 2	Time in Z 3	Time for Strength
M Plan										
Completed										
T Plan										
Completed										
W Plan										
Completed										
Th Plan										
Completed										
F Plan										
Completed										
S Plan										
Completed										
Su Plan										
Completed										

Target Hours This Week

Actual Hours This Week

Cumulative Training Hours

Drop cragging so that more time can be spent on Muscular Endurance training and alpine climbs.

CLIMBING NOTES

Date	_/_/_						_/_/_						_/_/_					
Vertical Gain																		
Grades																		
# of Pitches																		

STRENGTH TRAINING

Muscular Endurance	_/_/_	
	Lower Body	_____ Body
Distance		
Elevation +/-		
Time		
Weight		

Do 1 upper- and 1 lower-body Muscular Endurance workout if you are doing a technical climb, or do 2 Muscular Endurance lower-body workouts if you are doing a climb with low (for you) technical challenge. Make one of these a good one—try to exceed your previous efforts. No Max Strength or core workouts this week.

WEEKLY WORKOUT NOTES

	Grade	Workout Notes
M		
T		
W		
Th		
F		
S		
Su		

BASE PERIOD

DATE ____ / ____ / ____ **to** ____ / ____ / ____

> **!** You have almost done it! This is the last week of the Base Period and with a little more work you will be in the best shape of your life. Maintain the previous week's training distribution and volume. Mountaineers and alpinists alike will complete taxing Muscular Endurance and Max Strength workouts this week.
>
> 📖 P 223-253

WEEKLY TRAINING LOG

Activity by Time	Climb	Approach	Run	____	____	Altitude +/-	Time in Rec/Z 1	Time in Z 2	Time in Z 3	Time for Strength
M Plan										
Completed										
T Plan										
Completed										
W Plan										
Completed										
Th Plan										
Completed										
F Plan										
Completed										
S Plan										
Completed										
Su Plan										
Completed										

Target Hours This Week

Actual Hours This Week

Cumulative Training Hours

> 🧗 Drop cragging so that more time can be spent on Muscular Endurance training and alpine climbs.

CLIMBING NOTES

Date	__/__/__	__/__/__	__/__/__
Vertical Gain			
Grades			
# of Pitches			

STRENGTH TRAINING

Core Routine	_/_/_	
Exercise	Reps	Weight

Muscular Endurance	_/_/_	
	Lower Body	Upper Body
Distance		
Elevation +/-		
Time		
Weight		

 Do one complete Max Strength workout using the abbreviated core routine as your warm-up.

 On another day do 1 Muscular Endurance workout of your choice: upper or lower body.

Max Strength Routine	_/_/_	
Exercise	Reps	Weight
	/ / / / /	/ / / / /
	/ / / / /	/ / / / /
	/ / / / /	/ / / / /
	/ / / / /	/ / / / /

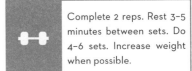 Complete 2 reps. Rest 3-5 minutes between sets. Do 4-6 sets. Increase weight when possible.

WEEKLY WORKOUT NOTES

	Grade	Workout Notes
M		
T		
W		
Th		
F		
S		
Su		

SPECIFIC PERIOD PLANNING

Utilizing the capacities you've built

This is the period where you convert all the preparatory fitness you have been building in the Base Period into the specific needs of the climb(s) you are gunning for. It will require significant imagination and input from you because this is where you tailor the training to fit your goals. Only you know what you are trying to accomplish, what your relative strengths and weaknesses are, and how much time you have. Be creative and have fun. Use the general guidelines laid out in the book rather than looking to the book for some magic formula or prescription.

Much of the training in this period will model the actual goal climb's physical requirements. The volume will drop, but the intensity of the climbing training sessions will increase, resulting in a jump in overall training load. Rest and recovery between these big sessions will become paramount because you need to be able to push yourself on these specific workouts and climbs in order to reap the full benefits. All other training done during this time will serve as maintenance. Once you build a particular physical quality it takes very little to maintain it. Max Strength and core workouts will be reduced in frequency and intensity to maintain, but not increase, the strength you have built. For some people with high strength, this can be as infrequently as one reduced workout every two weeks. Others may need a maintenance workout each week. For technical climbers these workouts might be done with an intense bouldering session in the gym or doing a few laps on a hard cragging route. Be sure to take long rests between laps to allow a near-max effort each time. Muscular Endurance work can easily be integrated into weekly alpine climbs for those that have access to real mountains. For those stuck in the flatlands, you will have to continue the weighted hill climbs by using the guidelines laid out in the book for progression of weight and vertical gain. All the systems that were stressed individually during the Base Period will be getting stressed jointly during the major workouts of this period. Much of the other work you do during this time will be geared toward simple recovery or light strength maintenance.

Refer back to chapter 9 in *Training for the New Alpinism* to help you plan this period. If you've laid a good foundation in the Base Period, you'll be able to achieve an extraordinarily high level of preparedness in four weeks.

Chapter 9

SPECIFIC PERIOD

DATE ____ / ____ / ____ to ____ / ____ / ____

> **!** Use 80% of the actual completed training volume from your last week of Base Period work as this week's target training volume. Consult page 265 for details of a mountaineering objective or page 268 for details of a technical climbing objective. Your training will concentrate on replicating the stresses of your climbing goal as much as possible given your circumstance.
>
> P 265 & P 268

WEEKLY TRAINING LOG

Activity by Time		Climb	Approach	Run	____	____	Altitude +/-	Time in Rec/Z 1	Time in Z 2	Time in Z 3	Time for Strength
M	Plan										
	Completed										
T	Plan										
	Completed										
W	Plan										
	Completed										
Th	Plan										
	Completed										
F	Plan										
	Completed										
S	Plan										
	Completed										
Su	Plan										
	Completed										

Target Hours This Week	
Actual Hours This Week	
Cumulative Training Hours	

CLIMBING NOTES

Date	_/_/_	_/_/_	_/_/_
Vertical Gain			
Grades			
# of Pitches			

STRENGTH TRAINING

Core Routine	_ / _ / _	
Exercise	Reps	Weight

Use a shortened core routine for maintenance during this period. It can be done as a warm-up for the shortened Max workouts. Doing 1 or 2 workouts every 2 weeks will be enough to maintain good strength for many weeks. Do 1–2 times through with 3–4 exercises done with near-maximum resistance.

Max Strength Routine	_ / _ / _	
Exercise	Reps	Weight

Mountaineers will want to continue with a gym-based Max Strength maintenance program of 1–2 workouts every 2 weeks. Technical alpinists can substitute maximum intensity climbing sessions for the weight room as strength maintenance.

Muscular Endurance	_ / _ / _
Distance	
Elevation +/-	
Time	
Weight	

All climbers will be able to substitute real approaches and climbs for the weighted hill climbs. If you don't have access to real mountains for this then continue doing laps with the water carries.

SPECIFIC

WEEKLY WORKOUT NOTES

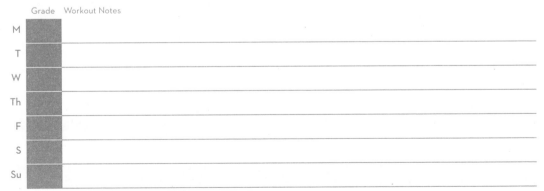

	Grade	Workout Notes
M		
T		
W		
Th		
F		
S		
Su		

SPECIFIC PERIOD

DATE _____ / _____ / _____ to _____ / _____ / _____

> **!** Use 75% of the actual completed training volume from your last week of Base Period work as this week's target training volume. Consult page 266 for details of a mountaineering objective or pages 268-269 for details of a technical climbing objective. Though your volume will drop these last weeks, the intensity and duration of individual bouts of exercise will increase. If the 2 big workouts this week don't take a mighty act of will to complete, they may be too easy.
>
> P 266 & P 268-269

WEEKLY TRAINING LOG

Activity by Time		Climb	Approach	Run	____	____	Altitude + / -	Time in Rec/Z 1	Time in Z 2	Time in Z 3	Time for Strength
M	Plan										
	Completed										
T	Plan										
	Completed										
W	Plan										
	Completed										
Th	Plan										
	Completed										
F	Plan										
	Completed										
S	Plan										
	Completed										
Su	Plan										
	Completed										

Target Hours This Week	
Actual Hours This Week	
Cumulative Training Hours	

CLIMBING NOTES

Date _ / _ / _   _ / _ / _   _ / _ / _

Vertical Gain															
Grades															
# of Pitches															

STRENGTH TRAINING

Core Routine	__ / __ / __	
Exercise	Reps	Weight

Use a shortened core routine for maintenance during this period. It can be done as a warm-up for the shortened Max workouts. Doing 1 or 2 workouts every 2 weeks will be enough to maintain good strength for many weeks. Do 1-2 times through with 3-4 exercises done with near-maximum resistance.

Max Strength Routine	__ / __ / __	
Exercise	Reps	Weight

Mountaineers will want to continue with a gym-based Max Strength maintenance program of 1-2 workouts every 2 weeks. Technical alpinists can substitute maximum intensity climbing sessions for the weight room as strength maintenance.

Muscular Endurance	__ / __ / __
Distance	
Elevation +/-	
Time	
Weight	

All climbers will be able to substitute real approaches and climbs for the weighted hill climbs. If you don't have access to real mountains for this then continue doing laps with the water carries.

SPECIFIC

WEEKLY WORKOUT NOTES

	Grade	Workout Notes
M		
T		
W		
Th		
F		
S		
Su		

SPECIFIC PERIOD

DATE _____ / _____ / _____ to _____ / _____ / _____

Use 70% of the actual completed training volume from your last week of Base Period work as this week's target training volume. Consult page 266 for details of a mountaineering objective or pages 269–270 for details of a technical climbing objective. These weeks require careful attention to recovery because the stress of the main workouts will be very high.

P 266 & P 269-270

WEEKLY TRAINING LOG

Activity by Time	Climb	Approach	Run	____	____	Altitude + / -	Time in Rec/Z 1	Time in Z 2	Time in Z 3	Time for Strength
M Plan										
Completed										
T Plan										
Completed										
W Plan										
Completed										
Th Plan										
Completed										
F Plan										
Completed										
S Plan										
Completed										
Su Plan										
Completed										

Target Hours This Week	
Actual Hours This Week	
Cumulative Training Hours	

CLIMBING NOTES

Date	__ / __ / __	__ / __ / __	__ / __ / __
Vertical Gain			
Grades			
# of Pitches			

STRENGTH TRAINING

Core Routine	__/__/__	
Exercise	Reps	Weight

Use a shortened core routine for maintenance during this period. It can be done as a warm-up for the shortened Max workouts. Doing 1 or 2 workouts every 2 weeks will be enough to maintain good strength for many weeks. Do 1–2 times through with 3–4 exercises done with near-maximum resistance.

Max Strength Routine	__/__/__	
Exercise	Reps	Weight

Mountaineers will want to continue with a gym-based Max Strength maintenance program of 1–2 workouts every 2 weeks. Technical alpinists can substitute maximum intensity climbing sessions for the weight room as strength maintenance.

Muscular Endurance	__/__/__
Distance	
Elevation +/-	
Time	
Weight	

All climbers will be able to substitute real approaches and climbs for the weighted hill climbs. If you don't have access to real mountains for this then continue doing laps with the water carries.

WEEKLY WORKOUT NOTES

	Grade	Workout Notes
M		
T		
W		
Th		
F		
S		
Su		

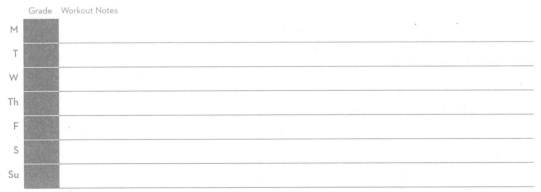
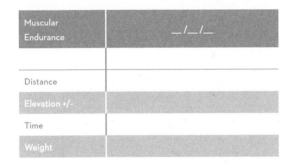

SPECIFIC PERIOD

DATE _____ / _____ / _____ to _____ / _____ / _____

> **!** Use 70% of the actual completed training volume from your last week of Base Period work as this week's target training volume. Consult page 266 for details of a mountaineering objective or pages 270–271 for details of a technical climbing objective. This is a consolidation week to allow this very high training load to be absorbed fully.
>
> P 266 & P 270-271

WEEKLY TRAINING LOG

Activity by Time		Climb	Approach	Run	____	____	Altitude +/-	Time in Rec/Z 1	Time in Z 2	Time in Z 3	Time for Strength
M	Plan										
	Completed										
T	Plan										
	Completed										
W	Plan										
	Completed										
Th	Plan										
	Completed										
F	Plan										
	Completed										
S	Plan										
	Completed										
Su	Plan										
	Completed										

Target Hours This Week	
Actual Hours This Week	
Cumulative Training Hours	

CLIMBING NOTES

Date	__/__/__	__/__/__	__/__/__
Vertical Gain			
Grades			
# of Pitches			

STRENGTH TRAINING

Core Routine	_/_/_	
Exercise	Reps	Weight

Use a shortened core routine for maintenance during this period. It can be done as a warm-up for the shortened Max workouts. Doing 1 or 2 workouts every 2 weeks will be enough to maintain good strength for many weeks. Do 1–2 times through with 3–4 exercises done with near-maximum resistance.

Max Strength Routine	_/_/_	
Exercise	Reps	Weight

Mountaineers will want to continue with a gym-based Max Strength maintenance program of 1–2 workouts every 2 weeks. Technical alpinists can substitute maximum intensity climbing sessions for the weight room as strength maintenance.

Muscular Endurance	_/_/_
Distance	
Elevation +/-	
Time	
Weight	

All climbers will be able to substitute real approaches and climbs for the weighted hill climbs. If you don't have access to real mountains for this then continue doing laps with the water carries.

SPECIFIC

WEEKLY WORKOUT NOTES

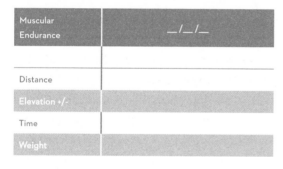

	Grade	Workout Notes
M		
T		
W		
Th		
F		
S		
Su		

TAPER PERIOD PLANNING

Ready or not

The training is now complete. The money is in the bank, so to speak. The goal during this period is to maintain your fitness and, most importantly, maintain your health. There is no more overreaching, no more capacity building. Now you need to dramatically reduce the training stress that your body has become accustomed to. If all the previous training has gone according to plan, this drop will give you a corresponding jump in fitness. During these weeks you should be feeling especially energetic and eager. Do not stop exercising, as this will make you feel sluggish and tired. But do not exert yourself to the levels that you were doing in the last few weeks of training.

You may be traveling a long distance to a foreign land. Take precautions to stay healthy or all the hard work of the previous year could be squandered. In the book we suggest appropriate volumes of maintenance workouts that do not push your capabilities, will keep you fit, and protect your health.

Chapter 10

Refer to chapter 10 in *Training for the New Alpinism* for guidance on planning this short period. Light maintenance training, especially of the aerobic type, will be all that is needed now.

TAPER PERIOD

DATE _____/_____/_____ to _____/_____/_____

> **!** Drop your training volume to half of last week's completed volume.

WEEKLY TRAINING LOG

Activity by Time	Climb	Approach	Run	___	___	Altitude +/-	Time in Rec/Z 1	Time in Z 2	Time in Z 3	Time for Strength
M Plan										
Completed										
T Plan										
Completed										
W Plan										
Completed										
Th Plan										
Completed										
F Plan										
Completed										
S Plan										
Completed										
Su Plan										
Completed										

Target Hours This Week	
Actual Hours This Week	
Cumulative Training Hours	

CLIMBING NOTES

Date	_/_/_	_/_/_	_/_/_
Vertical Gain			
Grades			
# of Pitches			

STRENGTH TRAINING

Core Routine	_/_/_	
Exercise	Reps	Weight

Max Strength Routine	_/_/_	
Exercise	Reps	Weight

During this period most people will want to do a single maintenance core workout, Max Strength workout, or Muscular Endurance workout once every 2 weeks.

Muscular Endurance	_/_/_
Distance	
Elevation +/-	
Time	
Weight	

WEEKLY WORKOUT NOTES

	Grade	Workout Notes
M		
T		
W		
Th		
F		
S		
Su		

TAPER

TAPER PERIOD

DATE _____ / _____ / _____ to _____ / _____ / _____

> ! Drop your training volume by 20% of last week's completed volume.

WEEKLY TRAINING LOG

Activity by Time		Climb	Approach	Run	____	____	Altitude +/-	Time in Rec/Z1	Time in Z2	Time in Z3	Time for Strength
M	Plan										
	Completed										
T	Plan										
	Completed										
W	Plan										
	Completed										
Th	Plan										
	Completed										
F	Plan										
	Completed										
S	Plan										
	Completed										
Su	Plan										
	Completed										

Target Hours This Week	
Actual Hours This Week	
Cumulative Training Hours	

CLIMBING NOTES

Date	_/_/_			_/_/_			_/_/_		
Vertical Gain									
Grades									
# of Pitches									

STRENGTH TRAINING

Core Routine	__ / __ / __	
Exercise	Reps	Weight

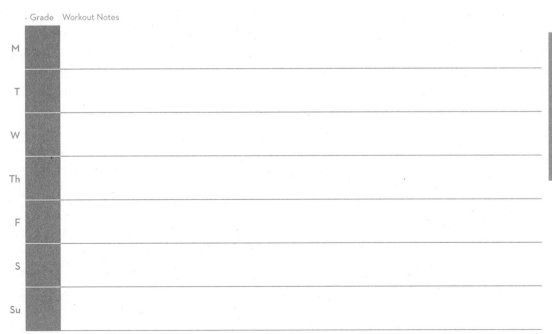

During this period most people will want to do a single maintenance core workout, Max Strength workout, or Muscular Endurance workout once every 2 weeks.

Max Strength Routine	__ / __ / __	
Exercise	Reps	Weight

Muscular Endurance	__ / __ / __
Distance	
Elevation +/-	
Time	
Weight	

WEEKLY WORKOUT NOTES

	Grade	Workout Notes
M		
T		
W		
Th		
F		
S		
Su		

TAPER

PEAK PERIOD PLANNING

You are a climbing machine

After months of building fitness and completing the Taper Period you should be ready to perform at a new personal-best level. The climbing you'll be doing during this period will replace any other training unless the breaks between climbs are more than one week. Then it can be advisable to toss in intermediate maintenance workouts. These can include such things as bouldering sessions as strength maintenance or runs for aerobic maintenance. You are a finely tuned climbing machine and your body thrives on exertion. Taking too long of a break from your routine will leave you feeling physically stale and flat.

Chapter 12

If you are going to be climbing at high altitude be sure to study chapter 12 in *Training for the New Alpinism*, which deals with altitude. The approach to base camp, living in base camp, and going high for acclimatization climbs are crucial to the success of your climb. We all have limited energy and it would be very unwise to go out of the starting gate too hard in the early days at a new altitude.

If you are planning a period of high-level climbing that is longer than five to six weeks, it is best to have a break of a couple of weeks in the middle to return to some basic training. This will allow you to regain the strength and endurance qualities that will have been lost during the previous intense climbing weeks. This usually means getting back into the gym for a Max Strength workout or doing a long mountain run at low intensity. Keep the aerobic volume high and the intensity low during this time. Eat well and focus on recovery. This change can extend a climbing season, and your top form, for another few weeks. If you've been hitting it hard, this break can be good mentally as well as physically.

We've carried forward the now familiar weekly training log, but stripped it of its usual headings. Here you can record whatever metric you like: vertical gain, grades of pitches, number of pitches, time in different heart-rate zones, etc. In our usage of such tables we've found these measures useful for future reference. Be liberal with your notes, having hard data about what you can physically accomplish now will inform not only your future training, but also your future climbing.

DATE _____/_____/_____ to _____/_____/_____

WEEKLY TRAINING LOG

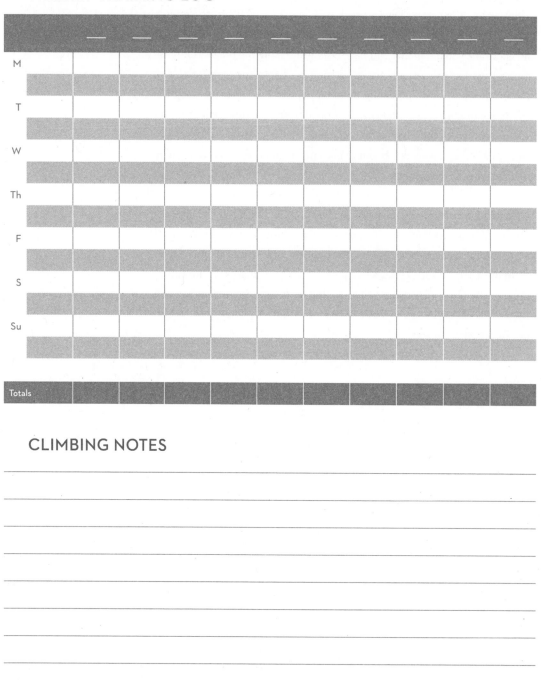

	—	—	—	—	—	—	—	—	—	—
M										
T										
W										
Th										
F										
S										
Su										
Totals										

CLIMBING NOTES

DATE _____ / _____ / _____ to _____ / _____ / _____

WEEKLY TRAINING LOG

	—	—	—	—	—	—	—	—	—	—
M										
T										
W										
Th										
F										
S										
Su										
Totals										

CLIMBING NOTES

_____
_____
_____
_____
_____
_____
_____
_____
_____

PEAK

DATE ____ / ____ / ____ to ____ / ____ / ____

WEEKLY TRAINING LOG

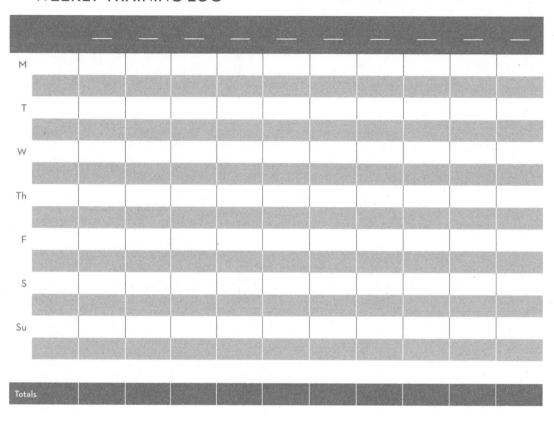

M											
T											
W											
Th											
F											
S											
Su											
Totals											

CLIMBING NOTES

_____

_____

_____

_____

_____

_____

_____

_____

_____

DATE ____/____/____ to ____/____/____

WEEKLY TRAINING LOG

	__	__	__	__	__	__	__	__	__	__
M										
T										
W										
Th										
F										
S										
Su										
Totals										

CLIMBING NOTES

_____

_____

_____

_____

_____

_____

_____

_____

PEAK

DATE ____ / ____ / ____ to ____ / ____ / ____

WEEKLY TRAINING LOG

	—	—	—	—	—	—	—	—	—	—	—
M											
T											
W											
Th											
F											
S											
Su											
Totals											

CLIMBING NOTES

_____

_____

_____

_____

_____

_____

_____

_____

_____

DATE _____/_____/_____ to _____/_____/_____

WEEKLY TRAINING LOG

	—	—	—	—	—	—	—	—	—	—
M										
T										
W										
Th										
F										
S										
Su										
Totals										

CLIMBING NOTES

_____

_____

_____

_____

_____

_____

_____

_____

_____

PEAK

DATE _____ / _____ / _____ to _____ / _____ / _____

WEEKLY TRAINING LOG

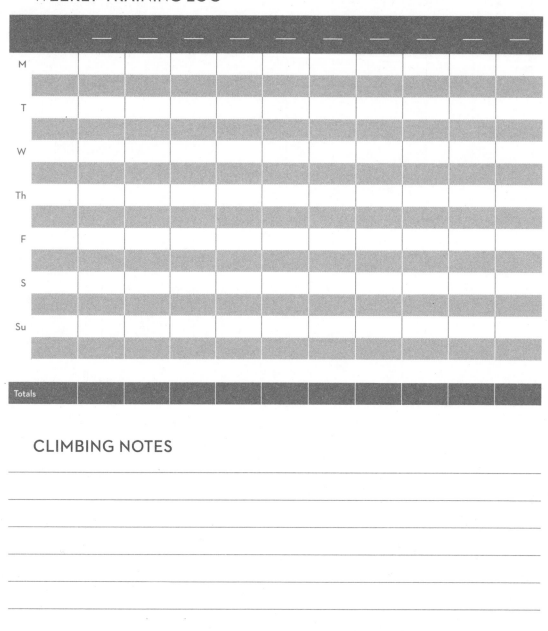

	—	—	—	—	—	—	—	—	—	—
M										
T										
W										
Th										
F										
S										
Su										
Totals										

CLIMBING NOTES

DATE _____ / _____ / _____ to _____ / _____ / _____

WEEKLY TRAINING LOG

	—	—	—	—	—	—	—	—	—	—
M										
T										
W										
Th										
F										
S										
Su										
Totals										

CLIMBING NOTES

_____

_____

_____

_____

_____

_____

_____

_____

_____

PEAK

DATE _____ / _____ / _____ to _____ / _____ / _____

WEEKLY TRAINING LOG

	—	—	—	—	—	—	—	—	—	—
M										
T										
W										
Th										
F										
S										
Su										
Totals										

CLIMBING NOTES

_____

_____

_____

_____

_____

_____

_____

_____

DATE ____ / ____ / ____ to ____ / ____ / ____

WEEKLY TRAINING LOG

	—	—	—	—	—	—	—	—	—	—
M										
T										
W										
Th										
F										
S										
Su										
Totals										

CLIMBING NOTES

_____

_____

_____

_____

_____

_____

_____

_____

_____

PEAK

APPENDIX

STRENGTH TRAINING NOTES

Since publication of *Training for the New Alpinism,* the most common questions from our readers have been about the application of strength training. Many people are confused by the roles of the different methods for training strength: general strength, Max Strength, and Muscular Endurance (ME) training. Many popular trainers and gyms targeting outdoor athletes advocate an overreliance on ME work that belies a serious misunderstanding of both coaching and physiology. As Mark Twight vividly describes in his essay "TINSTAAFL: There Is No Such Thing As A Free Lunch" (see page 94 in *Training for the New Alpinism*), the ME-heavy methods have very severe limitations in application to endurance sports. To help you guide your own training and to minimize the chance that you will diminish your training by getting sidetracked into sexy-sounding, but scientifically unsound training practices such as Cross-Fit and related ME-heavy methods, we have written

P 94

up a short, precise description of each form of strength training. It is our experience that once you understand the proper application of these three strength training methodologies you can apply them to any outdoor sport from bouldering and sport climbing to ski mountaineering and ultra-running.

Transitioning into Training: General Strength

Every year requires that you start with general strength (also called functional) training during your Transition Period. There are three important tasks you are aiming to accomplish during this time:

- **General strength.** Use a variety of whole-body movements involving a lot of different muscles to form a conditioning foundation for the Max Strength work to come. Remember that climbing-specific strength will be built upon whatever foundation of general strength you possess.

- **Flexibility.** We advocate movements that require a full range of motion that, by their nature, require flexibility. Flexibility and strength are closely related and what you perceive as a deficit in strength may in fact be a deficit in flexibility and vice versa.

- **Coordination.** Muscles that wire together, fire together. Improving neuromuscular connections is important for strength.

The functional hallmarks of general strength training are:

- **A strong and progressive core-strength component** to the training.

- **Ten repetitions of a movement** at roughly 50 to 60 percent of your one-rep maximum for that exercise.

- **Exercises performed in a circuit,** usually alternating between upper and lower body.

- **One to four circuits.**

- **Minimal rest.** Typically thirty seconds' rest between exercises and three minutes' rest between circuits to elicit a cardio-training effect.

- **Reliance on complex, multijoint exercises** that tax multiple muscle groups. Example: A barbell curl is a simple single-joint exercise, where as a pull-up is a complex movement that involves multiple joints.

Base Period Strength: Max Strength and Muscular Endurance

In the Base Period your goal is to build a strength reserve via Max Strength training and, once this is accomplished, convert that into muscular endurance. You have to build this in the correct order and there are no shortcuts. For a full discussion of the physiology of strength, reread chapters 4 and 5 of *Training for the New Alpinism*. Once the Base Period is complete, the rest of your year's strength training comes from maintenance workouts and doing your sport.

Chapters 4 & 5

Max Strength (Max)

In your Base Period we immediately introduce Max Strength training. This initial eight-week block of strength training will be focused on developing your maximum strength in two to four movements that use many of the major climbing muscles in a general way. It is best to pick one to two upper-body pushing/pulling exercises along with one to two lower-body lifting exercises.

The functional hallmarks of Max Strength training are:

- **Four repetitions at roughly 85** to **90 percent** of your one-rep maximum of that exercise.

- **Four to six sets.**

- **Three to five minutes** between sets to allow your muscles enough time to recover before another near-maximal effort.

- **Two to four movements** that are semispecific to climbing, such as pull-ups and box step-ups.

The time between lifts is important in order to allow for sufficient recovery and the completion of the four to six sets at the same or increasing weight. Many people get bored with all the rest in these workouts and will begin to hurry the workout and lose some of the effectiveness. If this applies to you, we recommend using a couplet system where you do a set of (for example) pull-ups, rest two minutes, then do a set of box step-ups, rest two minutes, and repeat the pull-ups. This compresses the workout without compromising its effect too much. You should not be pushing to failure on these sets. A well-executed Max Strength workout should leave you feeling energized, not wasted. If you're using the correct weight and getting really tired from these, reduce the number of sets.

Recall that a safe way of identifying your max lift (one-rep max) is to test yourself using a weight that allows three to five reps. If you can do three reps then that weight is close to 90 percent of your one-rep maximum, and if you can do five reps that weight is very close to 85 percent of your one-rep maximum. See page 229 of *Training for the New Alpinism* for more information.

P 229

Muscular Endurance (ME)

In the ninth week of the Base Period we introduce Muscular Endurance work mixed with Max Strength work that will continue to build over a twelve-week period. In a very real sense this is the training you've been preparing yourself to do. Once your strength reserve is (nearly) as high as it is going to get, you want to convert that strength into what is variously called power endurance (sometimes called strength endurance) or muscular endurance (sometimes called local muscular endurance). The difference between these terms is mainly one of duration with power endurance implying greater strength for shorter times. Power endurance is what many sport climbers train in their final phase of strength training. Alpinists are training their muscles to be able to maintain a high force output for hours rather than minutes.

Since the reason for the ME phase of training is to make you into a tireless climbing machine, you'll want to choose exercises as specific to climbing as you can dream up. If possible, actual climbing is your best bet. This follows the principle that all training starts general and becomes more and more specific as the athlete progresses. As with all strength training, once you understand the theory your imagination can be your guide. Though specificity (climbing) is ideal, this does not mean that you can't devise climbing-specific workouts to be done in a gym.

The functional hallmarks of lower-body Muscular Endurance training are:

- **Your rate of climb** should be limited by the fatigue felt in your legs, not your breathing.

- **Longer duration,** a minimum of 1,000 vertical feet of elevation gain.

- **Intensity is primarily in Zone 1.** Some Zone 3 ME sessions may be appropriate for the advanced athlete with multiple years of completed training.

- **Load and duration increase gradually** over the twelve-week period.

- **These workouts are very taxing** and require a minimum of seventy-two hours' rest between training bouts. Even for top athletes one of these sessions each week may be plenty.

- **You should feel dramatic improvements** from week to week. If you don't then you need more recovery between training sessions.

Because every alpine climb entails a lot of vertical gain, usually on steep ground, lower-body Muscular Endurance training is the cornerstone of our training program. To train our lower-body muscular endurance capacity we prefer to use steep uphill hiking and scrambling with and without added weight. The test of whether to add weight and if so, how much, is the following: If you can move fast enough that you cannot carry on a conversation, you need to add more weight to slow yourself down so that you are limited by your muscles' ability to use oxygen, not your heart's ability to supply it.

The functional hallmarks of upper-body Muscular Endurance training are:

- **Your ability to execute the exercise or movement** is limited by local muscular fatigue. A familiar example of this is forearm muscles becoming pumped to the point you fall off a rock or ice climb.

- **Longer duration of exercising,** whether the exercise is pull-ups or treadmill hand walking. This means at least one continuous minute for a minimum of two sets. (Sample progressions are given below.)

- **The duration increases gradually.**

- **These workouts are very taxing** and require a bare minimum of seventy-two hours of rest between training sessions. Even for top athletes one of these sessions each week may be plenty.

- **You should feel dramatic improvements** from week to week. If you don't then you need more recovery in between training sessions.

When you are doing upper-body ME workouts like treadmill hand walking or climbing, you should not be limited aerobically because the muscle mass engaged is much smaller. You should feel that the limitation is very much caused by localized muscular fatigue. If you are limited by breathing in these upper-body workouts, then you really need a lot more aerobic conditioning.

Exercise Variations

We often talk about the old standby exercises: pull-ups and dips for the upper body, and squats, deadlifts, and box step-ups for the lower body. Body weight works especially well for climbers training their upper body as it allows for the possibility of hanging weight from yourself. For the legs you'll be best served by using a barbell or a pack full of water or rocks as weight. Many variations of these exercises exist and imagination is the only limitation in finding one that suits your needs best. We've provided a list of variations that may help spur you to be more creative in your strength building. Each of these exercises are ones we've used or aspired to use and are listed in a progression from easy to hard. Many training books and online forums focus on strength exercises and their correct form.

Pull-Ups

Pull-ups can be executed on everything from a bar to ice tools. We prefer mixing our pull-ups between a bar and ice tools, gymnastic rings, or a towel hung over a bar. This seems to vary the movement pattern adequately so that, given a proper progression, joint issues are unlikely. Pull-ups, and any other body-weight exercises, are turned into Max Strength exercises by hanging weight off yourself. See our Special Strength Program for pull-ups on page 228 of *Training for the New Alpinism*. Note that if you cannot do one pull-up it may take you months of steady practice to get to that point, but once there additional gains will come much faster.

P 212–214 & P 228

- Chin-ups (palms facing you); use assistance, such as your toes on a chair, as necessary

- Pull-ups on a bar (palms facing away)

- Weighted pull-ups

- Wide-grip pull-ups

- Towel pull-ups

- Inclined two-arm pull-ups

- Campus ladder (see page 232 in *Training for the New Alpinism*)

P 232

- Typewriters

- Rope climb

- One-arm inclined pull-ups (see page 220–221 in *Training for the New Alpinism*)

P 220–221

- One-arm pull-up

- Front lever

- Front lever pull-ups

Dips

- Dips with your toes on a box

- Dips

- Parallel bar dips

- Ring dips

- Ring muscle up

- Bar muscle up

Squats

- Air front squat (no bar or wooden bar)

- Goblet squat

- Weighted front squat

- Back squat

- Overhead squat (perhaps our favorite for climbers due to core and shoulder involvement)

- Single-leg squat

- Hang clean with deep catch to front squat

Deadlifts

- Romanian or straight-leg deadlift

- Single-leg straight-leg deadlift

- Conventional deadlift

- Clean

- Clean and jerk

Box Step-Ups

- Side step-up (quadriceps dominant)

- Side step-down (quadriceps dominant)

- Front step-up (hamstring/gluteus dominant, most specific)

- Front step-down (very quadriceps dominant)

Lower-Body Muscular Endurance Exercises

P 234-239

A proven method that we have used many times is hiking uphill with jugs of water. Refer to pages 234–239 in *Training for the New Alpinism* for a complete discussion. The amount of weight you use is completely dependent upon the aerobic capacity of the muscle fibers needed to get your body plus additional weight up the climb. Author Steve House has been able to use as much as forty-two pounds and cover 4,000 feet in these workouts. There is no single recipe that fits everyone, so it will be helpful for you to think about the big days on your goal climb. If that entails a day of 3,000 vertical feet with fifty pounds at high altitude then you darned well better be exceeding that in your training at lower elevation. Start with 50 percent of your goal-climb's vertical with 0 to 50 percent of the weight you'll carry on that climb.

As an example of adding variety to this type of workout, before heading to climb K7 in Pakistan Steve used a fun, easy route called the South Arête of South Early Winter Spire, which is 700 feet long and rated 5.6. One approach to this climb is a 2,000-foot steep snow gully. Steve booted up this gully and then did six to twelve laps climbing up and down the South Arête as an ME workout. His typical time to climb the route was eight minutes. These workouts were not only effective, but they were fun and inspiring.

Upper-Body Muscular Endurance Exercises

Most of us will not need added weight for these upper-body ME workouts. Here are several excellent applications of these training techniques that are highly climbing specific.

1   **Multiple laps** (possibly climbing up and down) on a sport route, ice climb, bouldering traverse, one to two number grades below your on-sight ability so that you are climbing continuously for twenty minutes. Start with one rep. When you can do three reps, add 10 percent of your body weight and start the process over. A Treadwall is a perfect device for training upper-body muscular endurance. Refer back to the principles explained above and on pages 233–241 of *Training for the New Alpinism*.

P 233–241

2   **Treadmill hand walking.** Start with five sets of one minute of walking with two minutes' rest. Use this progression when you achieve each new level:

- 5x1' w/2' rest until you can progress to next level

- 5x1' w/1' rest until you can progress to next level

- 10x1' w/2' rest until you can progress to next level

- 3x5x2' w/2' rest and 5' between sets until you can progress to next level

- 2x5x3' w/1' rest and 5' between sets

3   **Gym climb or at the crag Muscular Endurance training.** This exercise can be done in a gym or on an easily top-roped rock or ice climb. Start by climbing continuously for one repetition of five to ten minutes on routes that are difficult enough to elicit the sensation of a pump in localized muscles such as upper body or forearms, but not so hard that you pump out and fall off. The reason we recommend doing this on top-rope is so that you can move more continuously. Be sure to stop before failure. Switch with a climbing partner who does the same thing. Do this once per week for the first two weeks and in the third week start adding additional repetitions that are 50 percent as long as your first repetition. We'll fill out the example with the five-minute session:

- 5'x1, equal amounts of rest

- 5'x1, equal amounts of rest

- 5'x1, 2.5'x1, equal amounts of rest

- 5'x1, 2.5'x1, 2.5'x1, equal amounts of rest

- 5'x1, 5'x1, equal amounts of rest

- 5'x1, 5'x1, 2.5'x1, equal amounts of rest

- 5'x1, 5'x1, 2.5'x1, 2.5'x1, equal amounts of rest

- 5'x1, 5'x1, 5'x1, equal amounts of rest

- 5'x1, 5'x1, 5'x1, 2.5'x1, equal amounts of rest

- 5'x1, 5'x1, 5'x1, 2.5'x1, 2.5'x1, equal amounts of rest

- 5'x1, 5'x1, 5'x1, 5'x1, equal amounts of rest

- 5'x1, 5'x1, 5'x1, 5'x1, 5'x1, equal amounts of rest

If you are able to do the above week's 10, 11, or 12 workouts, then you need to climb more difficult and/or sustained routes or add weight until you can elicit a steady pump with five to ten minutes of climbing time.

If you feel yourself regressing from one Muscular Endurance workout to another, it means you are not recovered and you need more rest between workouts. Or you may be climbing too much or too hard outside. Recovery has to be long enough to allow progression or you will become overtrained.

Some of our most rewarding training days have been when we used our imagination to create fun, challenging, and progressive Muscular Endurance workouts. Because this work is so physically demanding you don't want it to be a drag mentally.

REFERENCE DIAGRAMS FOR SCOTT'S KILLER CORE ROUTINE

STRICT SIT-UPS

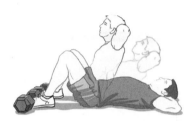

BIRD DOGS

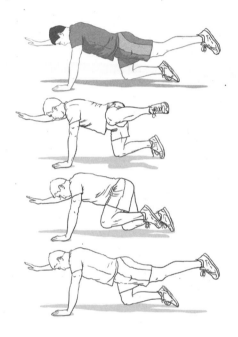

WINDSHIELD WIPERS

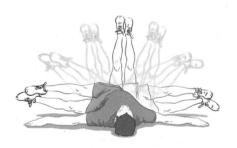

THREE-P/TWO-POINT PLANKS

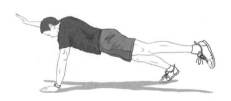

KAYAKERS

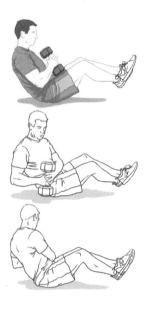

SUPER PUSH-UPS

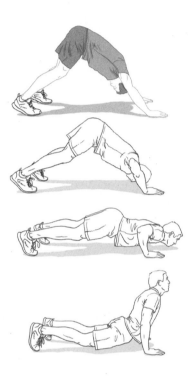

HANGING LEG RAISES

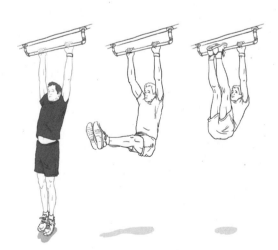

BRIDGES

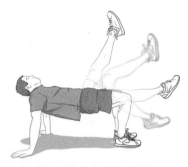

GYMNASTIC L-SITS

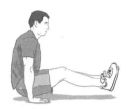

SIDE PLANKS

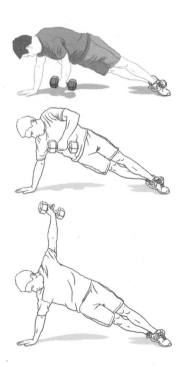